ENDOMORPH DIET FOR BEGINNERS

THE COMPLETE GUIDE TO BURN FAT AND LOSE WEIGHT WITH DELICIOUS RECIPES & EXERCISE PLAN

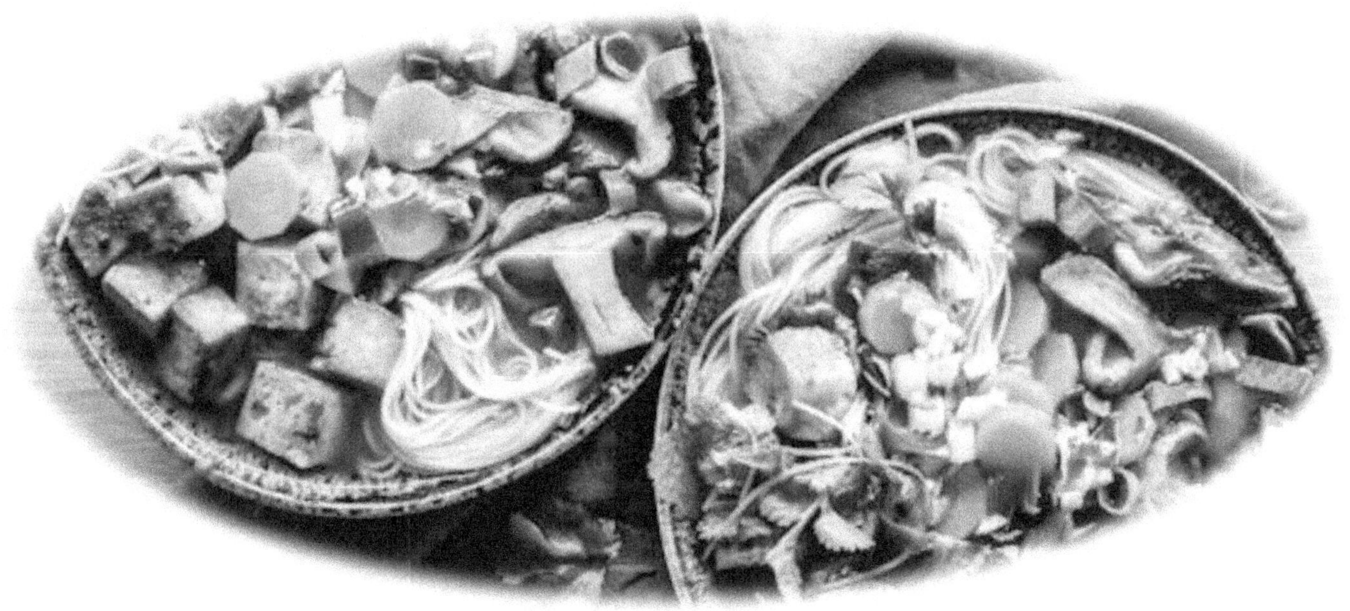

KEVIN S. MAXWELL

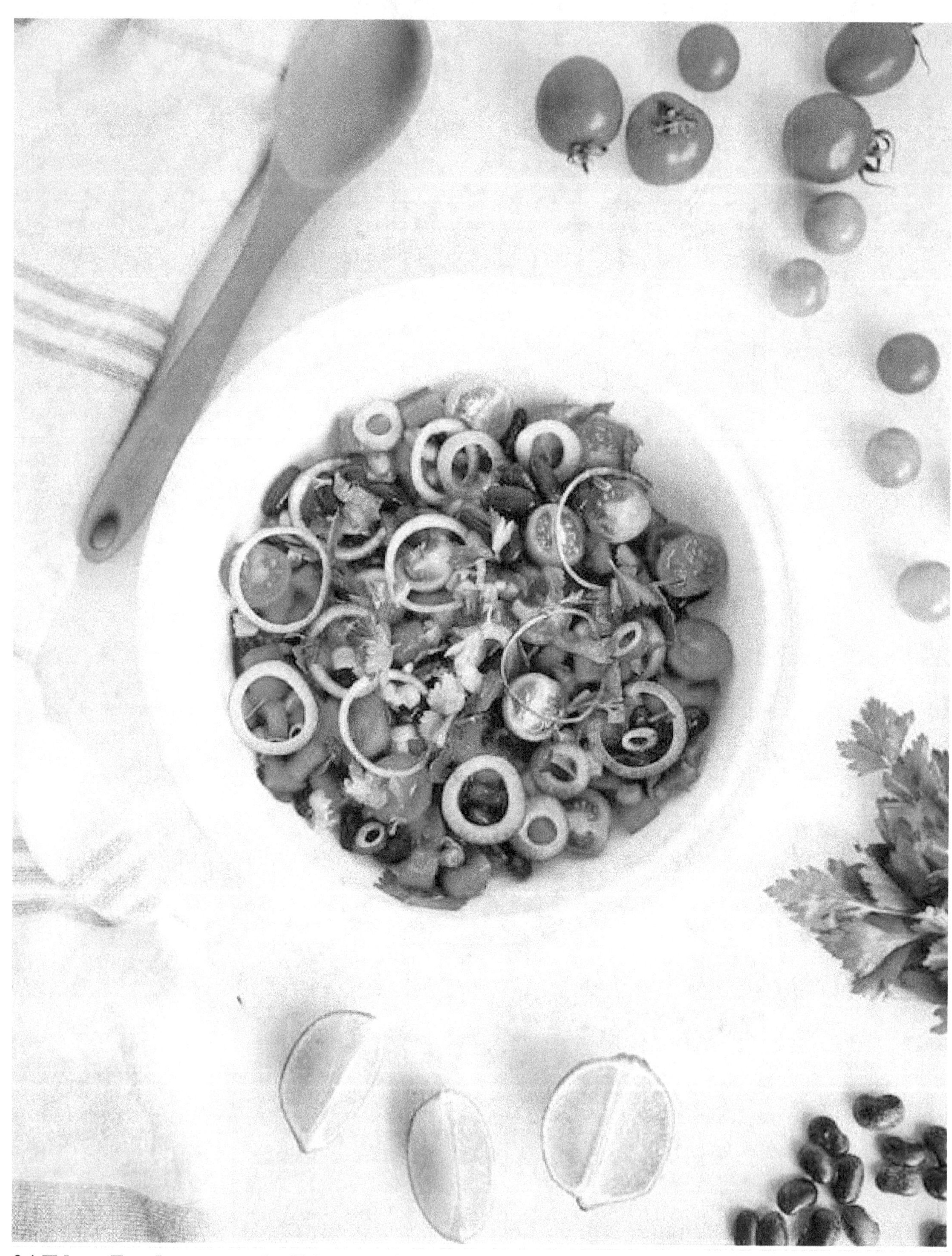

Copyright © 2024 by Kevin S. Maxwell

EMAIL ME!

I know that exploring topics that involve food and nutrition can often lead to questions and uncertainty. I invite you to contact me with any questions you may have. I'm here to assist.

Please contact me through email at **kevinmaxwelldiet@gmail.com**, and I will try my best to respond to you within 24 hours.

HOW TO USE THIS COOKBOOK

❖ **Browse Recipes:** Start by exploring through the cookbook and examining the many recipes offered. There are suggestions for every mealtime, from breakfast to lunch, dinner, and snacks.

❖ **Choose Your Meals:** Select meals that appeal to you and are consistent with your nutritional choices and objectives. Whether you want a robust salad, a soothing stir-fry, or a quick snack, there are alternatives to fit everyone's taste.

❖ **Plan Your Week:** Take some time to plan your meals for the next week. Consider convenience, ingredients on hand, and any special occasions or events that may impact your meal selection.

❖ **Shop for supplies:** Create a shopping list based on the recipes you've selected, making sure you have all of the supplies on hand. Choose fresh, healthful foods wherever feasible, and consider storing up on pantry staples to make meal preparation easier.

❖ **Prepare and enjoy:** Follow the cookbook's step-by-step directions to easily create each meal. Enjoy creating and eating homemade meals, knowing that you're fueling your body with tasty and healthy foods. Continue the approach each week to get the advantages of this endomorph-friendly diet.

Table of CONTENT

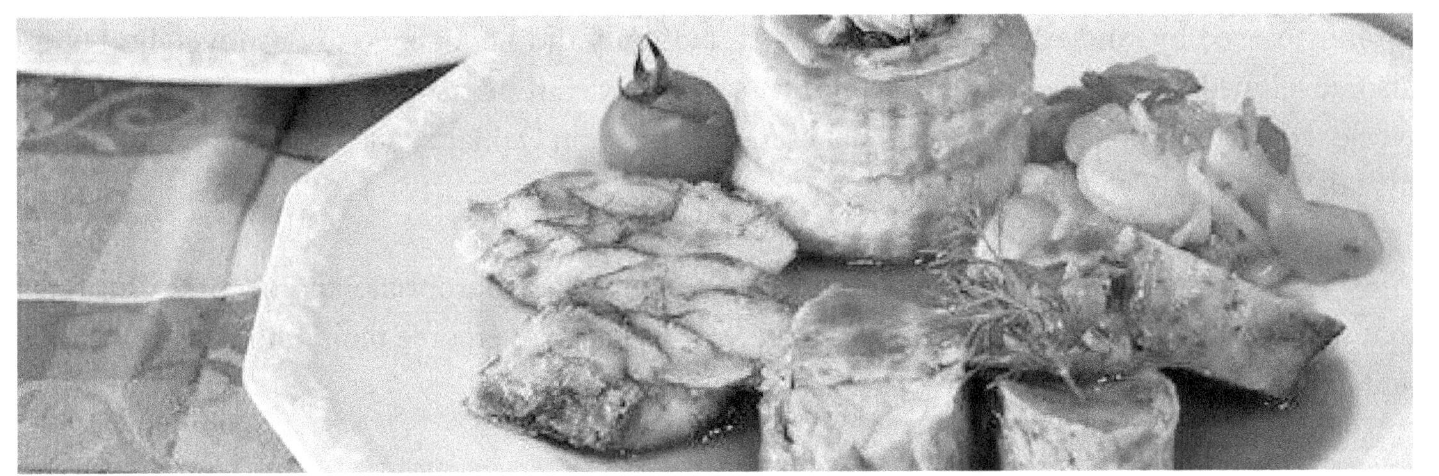

INTRODUCTION

There was an elderly man called Alex who resided in the lively city of Oakland. Alex, a retired educator, was well-known for his cheery personality and his passion for telling stories. He had always been renowned for these qualities. Nevertheless, as time went on, Alex became aware that his body was not nearly as nimble as it had been in the past. The roundness and softness of his body had increased, and his energy levels had decreased. He was advised by his physician that he had an endomorph body type, which indicated that he had a slower metabolism and a natural tendency to retain fat, particularly around the waist.

Alex was certain that he would choose not to let his physical appearance influence his health. With the help of the appropriate diet and exercise routine that was designed specifically for his endomorphic physique, he set out on a path to control his weight. After consulting with Amada, a nutritionist, he was recommended to follow a diet that would lower the number of calories he consumed while simultaneously boosting the intake of lean proteins, healthy fats such as omega fatty acids, and low carbohydrates[1]. She stressed the need to avoid processed carbohydrates and concentrate on healthy meals such as salmon, asparagus, and leafy greens to achieve optimal health.

In addition to his diet, Alex began an exercise routine that includes high-intensity interval training to enhance his cardiovascular health[3] and strength training to develop muscle, which burns more calories than fat as a source of energy. He also took care to enhance his non-exercise activity thermogenesis by taking quick walks around the neighborhood and gardening, activities he found pleasurable and sustainable.

Months passed by, and Alex's efforts paid off. Not only did he manage to drop weight, but he also developed muscle and vigor. He felt like a new guy, full of energy and ready to take on the world. His metamorphosis became an inspiration to many in Oakland, and he would regularly tell his tale to anybody willing to listen.

Alex's tale is a testimony to the power of dedication and the appropriate approach. It illustrates that with the right information and a little work, anybody can overcome their inherent inclinations and enjoy a better, happier life.

And so, Alex lived out his days, not only as a storyteller but as a living example of how the appropriate diet and exercise regimen can improve a life, particularly for individuals with an endomorphic body type. That is what this cookbook would guide you on.

CHAPTER ONE

WHAT IS AN ENDOMORPH

The endomorph body type is one of the three basic somatotypes, characterized by a rounder physique, bigger bone structure, and a predisposition to retain fat, notably around the lower belly, hips, and thighs. Endomorphs frequently have a smooth and curvaceous look with a broad waist and hips. They tend to have a larger proportion of body fat and muscle, which may make weight control a challenge.

Endomorphs are known to have a slower metabolism, which means they burn calories at a slower pace compared to other body types. This might lead to weight gain if their food and exercise levels are not adequately maintained. To combat this, endomorphs may benefit from a customized diet plan that focuses on reduced carbohydrate consumption and greater protein and healthy fats, which may assist in increasing satiety and maintaining muscle maintenance.

When it comes to exercise, endomorphs need to participate in regular physical activity to enhance their metabolism and encourage weight reduction. A mix of aerobic workouts, such as jogging or cycling, and strength training may be especially helpful. Cardio helps to burn calories and enhance heart health, while strength training develops muscle, which may boost the body's resting metabolic rate.

High-intensity interval training (HIIT) is also advised for endomorphs since it may give a more effective exercise by combining brief bursts of intense activity with periods of relaxation. This sort of exercise may assist in burning a substantial quantity of calories in a shorter time and may also enhance insulin sensitivity, which is excellent for weight management.

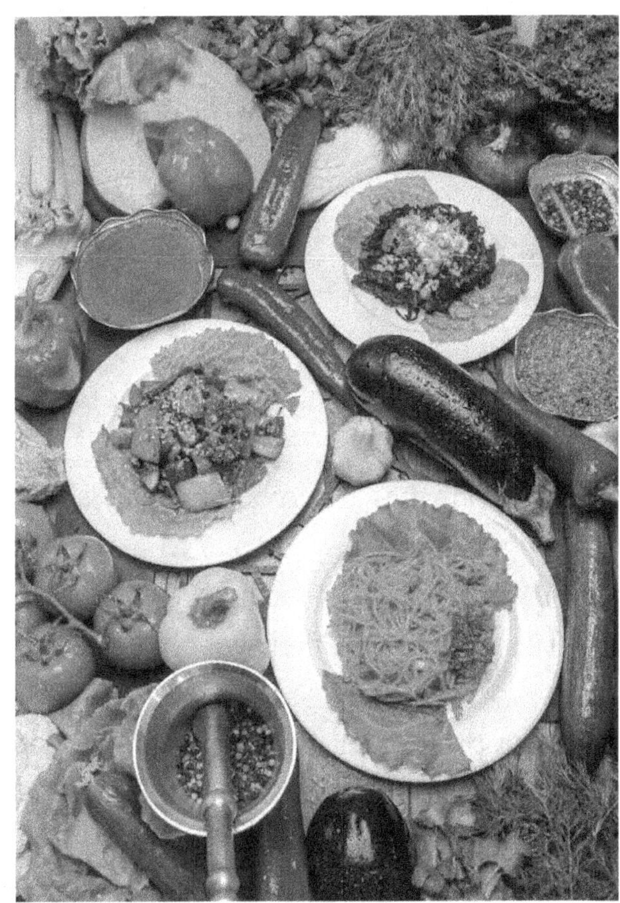

In addition to exercise, lifestyle adjustments such as increasing daily mobility and minimizing sedentary habits may also benefit endomorphs in regulating their weight. Activities like walking, using the stairs instead of the elevator, and standing more frequently during the day may lead to a greater daily calorie expenditure.

Endomorphs must recognize that although they may be inclined to certain physical features, with the correct diet and exercise regimen, they may reach their health and fitness objectives. It's about finding a sustainable technique that works for their body shape and sticking to it consistently.

Overall, the endomorph body type demands a thoughtful approach to nutrition and activity. By concentrating on nutritious meals, participating in regular physical exercise, and adopting good lifestyle choices, endomorphs may successfully control their weight and enhance their overall health.

UNDERSTANDING ENDOMORPH BODY TYPE

Understanding the endomorph body type includes identifying the particular physical traits and metabolic problems associated with this somatotype. Endomorphs are often characterized by a larger physique, with a predisposition to accumulate fat more quickly than other body types. They frequently have a rounder shape, with a broad waist and robust bone structure.

The notion of somatotypes, including the endomorph body type, was presented by psychologist William H. Sheldon. According to his idea, endomorphs have a larger percentage of body fat and muscle, which might make it hard to reduce weight. However, this body shape is not always linked with obesity; it's more about the natural distribution of fat and muscle.

Endomorphs may discover that they acquire weight readily, particularly in the lower belly, hips, and thighs. This may be due to a slower metabolism, which means calories are expended at a slower pace. As a consequence, endomorphs need to be extra aware of their food and exercise routines to maintain their weight effectively.

An appropriate diet for an endomorph often comprises a reduced amount of carbs and a greater intake of proteins and healthy fats. This dietary strategy helps to improve satiety and retain muscle mass while regulating calorie intake. It's also vital for endomorphs to concentrate on natural meals and avoid processed and refined carbs that might contribute to weight gain2.

Exercise is equally vital for endomorphs. A mix of aerobic activities and strength training may assist enhance metabolism and promote fat reduction. High-intensity interval training (HIIT) is especially advantageous since it delivers a tough exercise that may burn a considerable number of calories in a short time. Regular physical exercise is crucial for endomorphs to increase their metabolism and maintain a healthy weight.

Endomorphs need to recognize that although they may tend a specific body type, with the correct lifestyle modifications, including food and exercise, they may reach their health and fitness objectives. Consistency and a personalized approach to diet and physical exercise are crucial to controlling the endomorph body type properly.

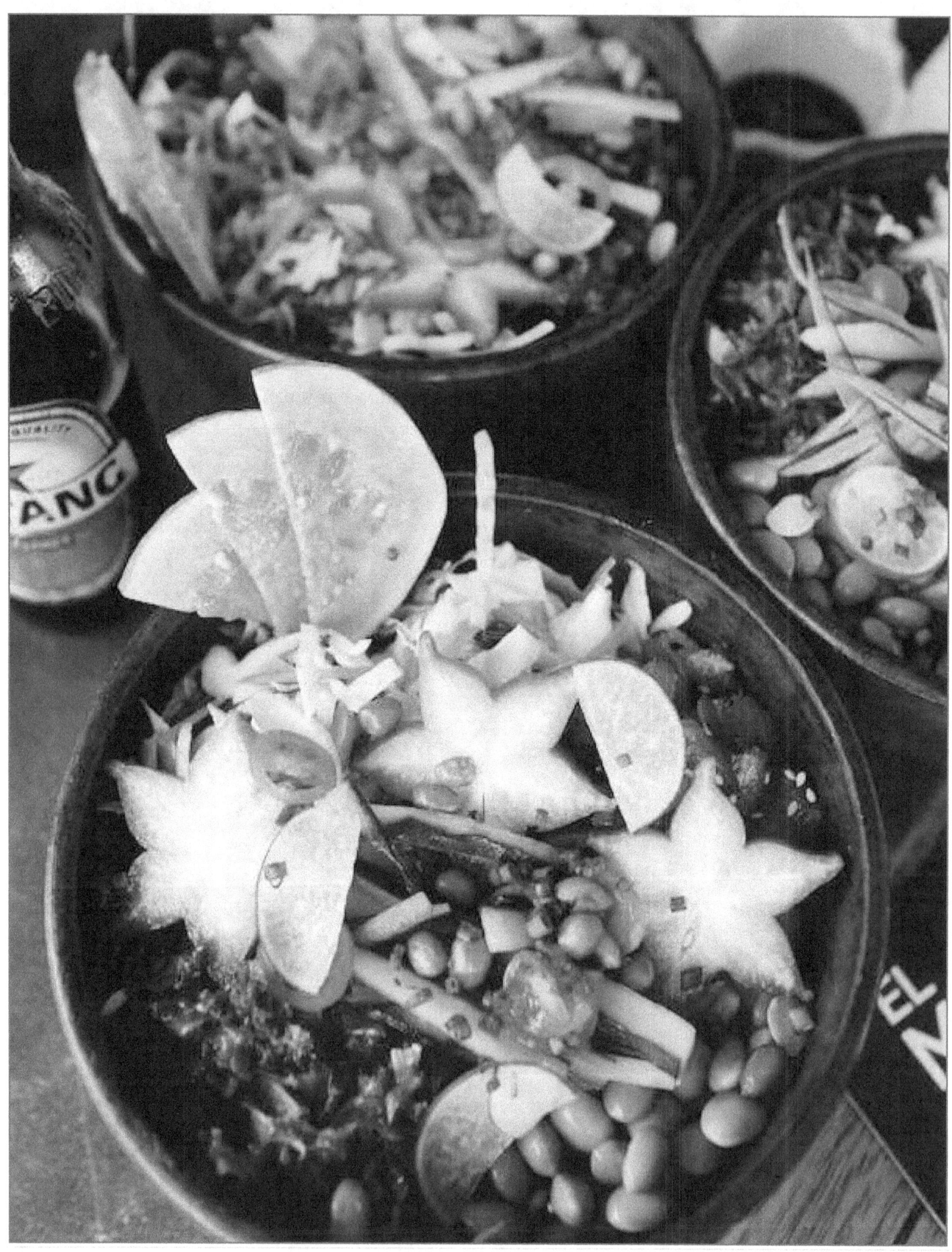

CHAPTER TWO

UNDERSTANDING ENDOMORPH DIET

The Endomorph Diet is especially developed for persons with an endomorphic body type, which is characterized by a greater inclination to retain fat, particularly around the waist. This body type generally suffers from a sluggish metabolism, making weight control a challenge.

Concerning the Endomorph Diet, the emphasis is on a balanced intake of macronutrients that aid weight reduction and muscle maintenance. The diet often includes a decrease in carbohydrates, particularly processed carbs, and an increase in protein and healthy fats. This helps to control insulin sensitivity, which is critical for endomorphs since they tend to be more prone to insulin resistance.

Protein-rich diets like lean meats, fish, and eggs are prioritized to help grow and sustain muscle mass. Healthy fats from sources such as avocados, almonds, and olive oil are suggested to enhance satiety and offer energy. Complex carbs are given but in moderation, concentrating on vegetables and nutritious grains to minimize blood sugar spikes.

The fitness regimen for endomorphs often involves a combination of strength training and aerobic routines. Strength training is vital for growing muscle, which may boost the resting metabolic rate and help in weight reduction. Cardiovascular workouts, such as jogging or cycling, assist to burn calories and enhance heart health. High-Intensity Interval Training (HIIT) is also advised since it may lead to more effective calorie burning in a shorter period.

Together, the Endomorph Diet and activity plan seek to establish a calorie deficit while maintaining metabolic health, leading to sustained weight reduction and better body composition for persons with an endomorphic body type.

BENEFITS OF ENDOMORPH DIET

The advantages of the Endomorph Diet are customized to meet the special demands of persons with an endomorphic body type.

Here are several significant advantages:

Weight Loss: The diet is intended to assist endomorphs lose weight by producing a calorie deficit via a balanced intake of macronutrients.

High Energy Levels: A concentration of proteins and vitamins ensures that endomorphs retain higher energy levels, which is crucial for their slower metabolism.

Muscle Building: High protein intake encourages muscle growth, which can help in burning stored fat and improving body composition.

Improved Health: The diet emphasizes a healthy approach to food, promoting overall well-being and balance.

Improved Lifestyle: By adopting the Endomorph Diet, individuals may experience a positive shift in their lifestyle, leading to better health habits and choices.

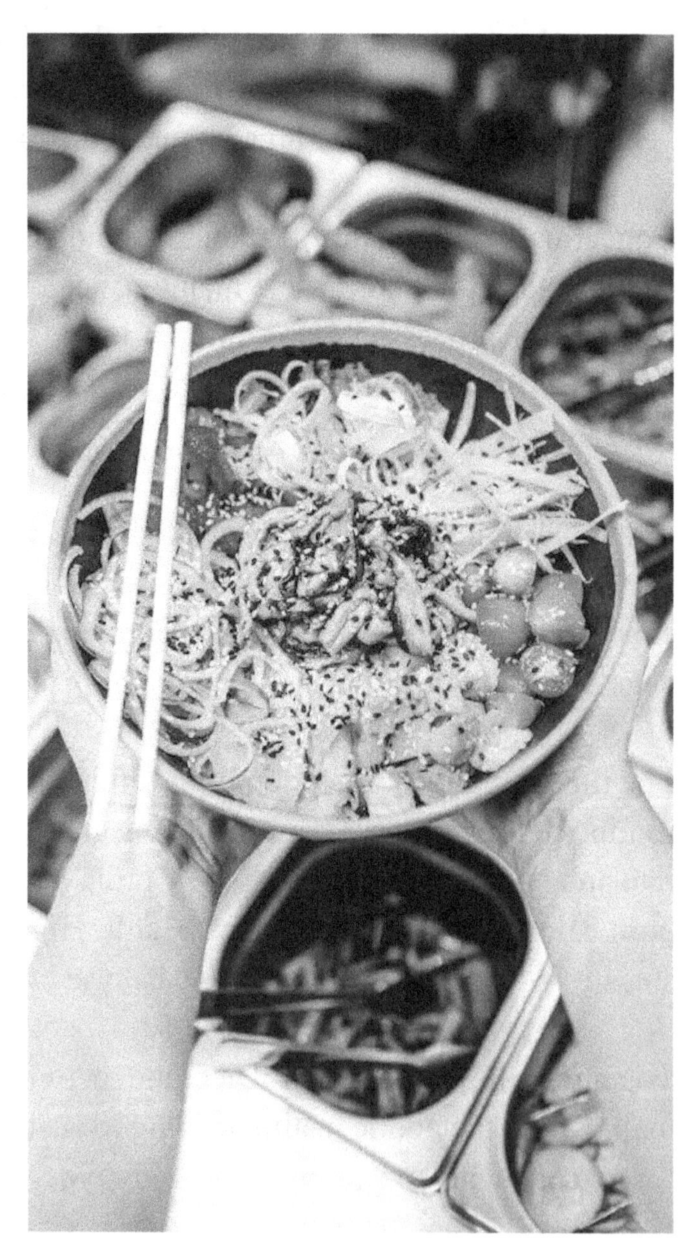

TIPS TO ACHIEVE OPTIMAL HEALTH WITH ENDOMORPH DIET

For people with an endomorphic body type, obtaining maximum health via nutrition needs a deliberate approach to food selections. Here's a tip on what to eat and what to avoid:

Foods to Eat

1. **Lean Proteins:** opt for chicken, turkey, and fish to build muscle and promote satiety.
2. **Healthy Fats:** Include sources like avocados, nuts, and olive oil for energy and fullness.
3. **Fiber-Rich Vegetables:** Consume a variety of vegetables to aid digestion and maintain fullness.
4. **Complex Carbohydrates:** Choose whole grains and legumes in moderation to manage insulin sensitivity.
5. **Low Glycemic Fruits:** Berries and apples are good options for their fiber content and lower sugar impact.

Foods to Avoid

1. **Refined Carbohydrates:** Limit white bread, spaghetti, and sugary snacks that may boost blood sugar levels.
2. **Processed Meats:** Avoid fatty cuts of meat and processed choices like bacon, which are rich in harmful fats.
3. **High-Sugar Foods:** Stay away from sweets and sugary beverages that promote fat storage.
4. **High-Fat Dairy:** Full-fat yogurt and cheese may be calorie-dense and should be taken in moderation.

In combination with the diet, an exercise plan for endomorphs should incorporate strength training to develop muscle and aerobic routines to burn fat. High-Intensity Interval Training (HIIT) is also useful for its effectiveness in calorie burning and boosting cardiovascular health4. By combining these food suggestions with a steady exercise plan, endomorphs may strive towards reaching and maintaining maximum health. Remember, the key is balance and consistency in both nutrition and activity.

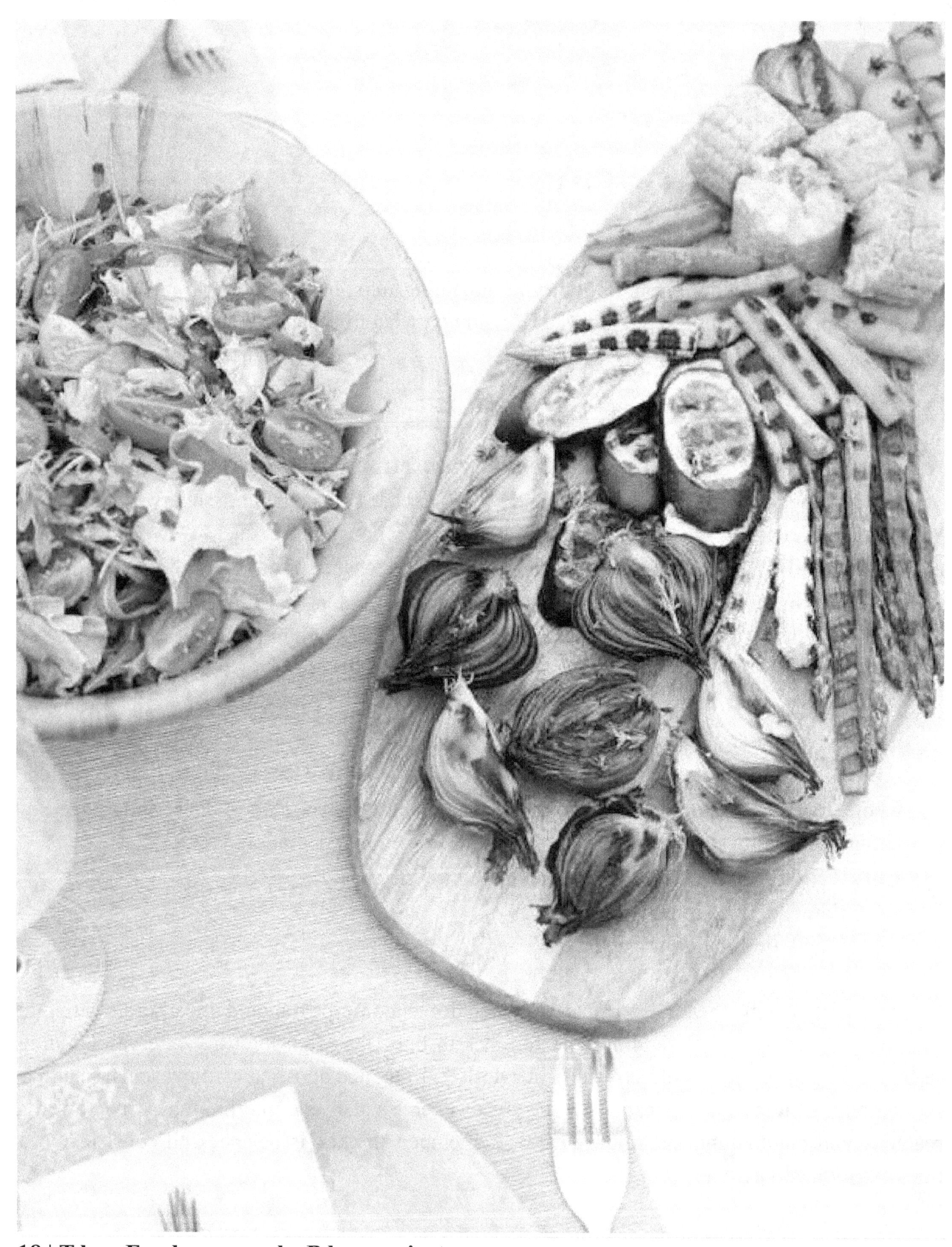

CHAPTER THREE

LIST OF INGREDIENTS

Here's a healthy shopping list based on the recipes provided:

Proteins

- Chicken breasts
- Turkey breast slices
- Salmon fillets
- Lean ground turkey
- Eggs
- Greek yogurt
- Cottage cheese
- Canned tuna
- Firm tofu
- Shrimp

Vegetables

- Spinach
- Mixed greens (lettuce, arugula)
- Asparagus
- Broccoli
- Bell peppers
- Zucchini
- Cauliflower
- Kale
- Eggplant
- Cherry tomatoes
- Cucumber

Fruits

- Berries (strawberries, blueberries, raspberries)
- Avocado
- Lemons
- Apples
- Pineapple

Healthy Fats

- Olive oil
- Almond butter
- Nuts (almonds, walnuts)
- Seeds (chia seeds, flaxseeds)

Carbohydrates

- Quinoa
- Whole-grain bread
- Whole-grain tortillas
- Brown rice or cauliflower rice
- Sweet potatoes
- Oats

Dairy and Dairy Alternatives

- Almond milk
- Parmesan cheese
- Feta cheese

Herbs, Spices, and Condiments

- Garlic
- Fresh herbs (thyme, rosemary, parsley, dill)
- Soy sauce
- Balsamic vinegar
- Lemon juice
- Basil pesto
- Marinara sauce
- Chili powder
- Cumin
- Red pepper flakes

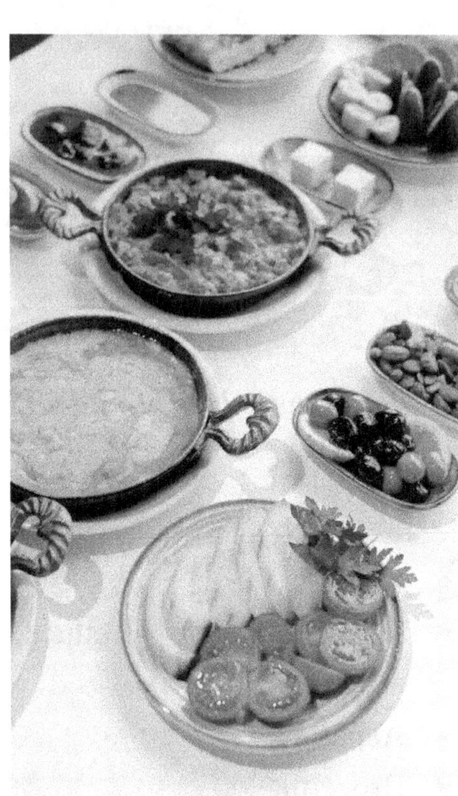

Miscellaneous

- Hummus
- Greek yogurt (plain)
- Dijon mustard
- Vinegar (for poaching eggs)
- Protein powder (optional for smoothies and pancakes)

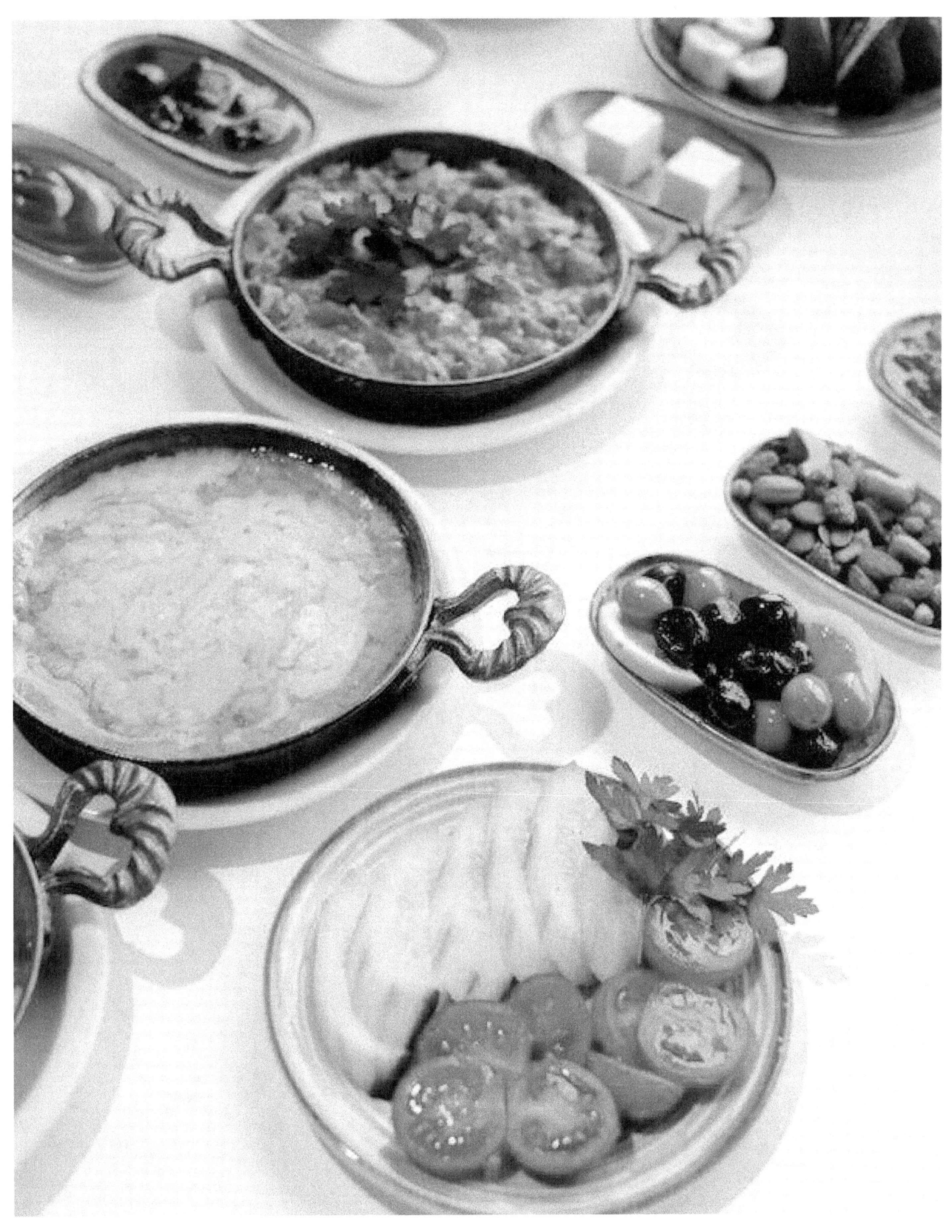

CHAPTER FOUR
BREAKFAST RECIPES

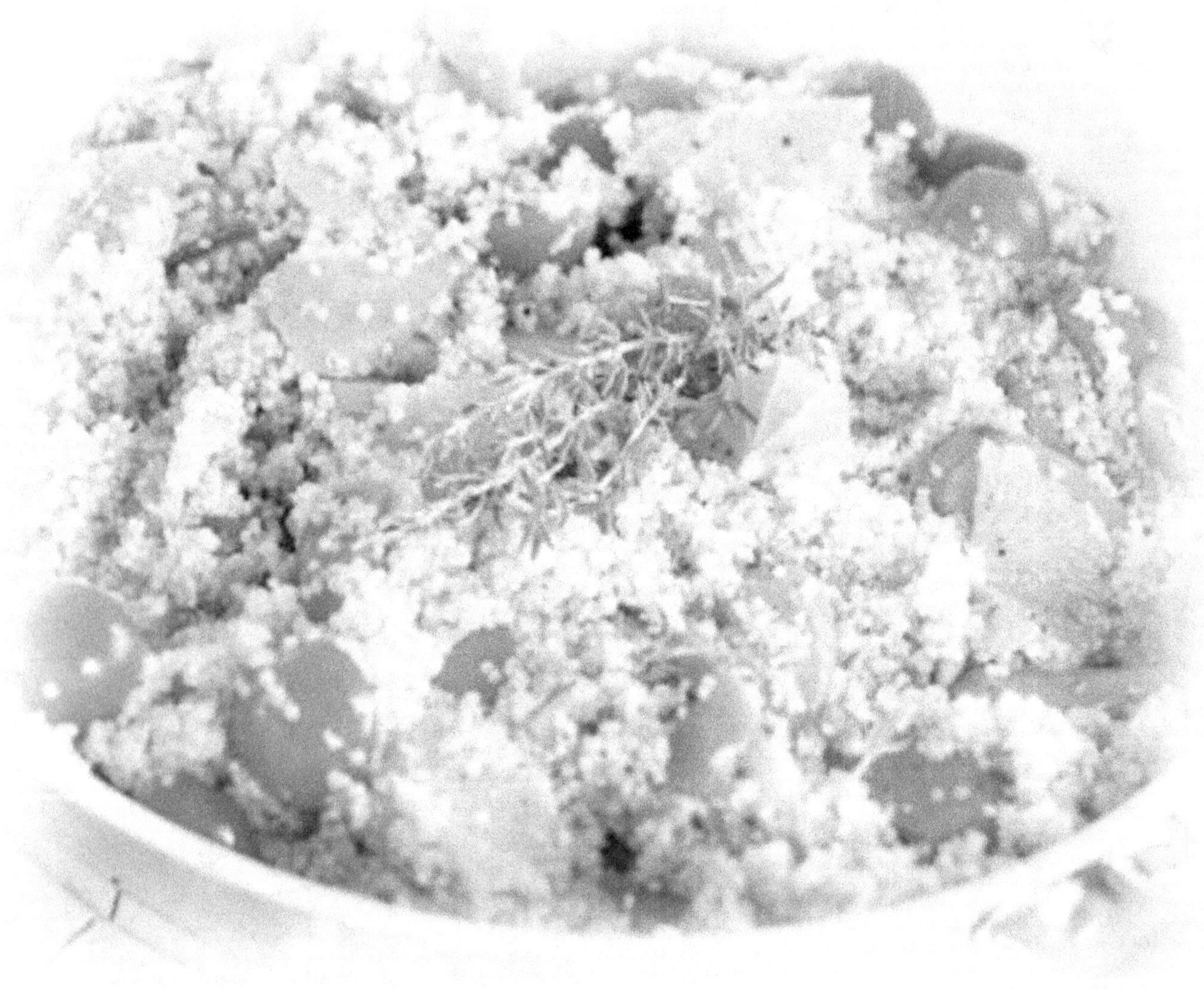

Spinach and Mushroom Omelette

- ➤ 2 eggs
- ➤ 1 cup spinach, fresh
- ➤ 1/2 cup mushrooms, sliced
- ➤ 1 tbsp olive oil
- ➤ Salt and pepper to taste

DIRECTIONS

- ✓ Heat olive oil in a non-stick pan over medium heat.
- ✓ Sauté mushrooms until they're soft.
- ✓ Add spinach and cook until wilted.
- ✓ Beat the eggs and pour over the vegetables in the pan.
- ✓ Cook until the eggs are set on the bottom, then fold the omelet in half.
- ✓ Serve hot with a sprinkle of salt and pepper.

Avocado Toast with Poached Egg

- 1 slice of whole-grain bread
- 1/2 ripe avocado
- 1 egg
- 1 tsp vinegar
- Salt and pepper to taste

DIRECTIONS

- ✓ Toast the bread to your liking.
- ✓ Mash the avocado and spread it on the toast.
- ✓ Bring water to a simmer in a pot and add vinegar.
- ✓ Crack the egg into a cup and gently pour it into the simmering water.
- ✓ Poach the egg for 3-4 minutes, then remove with a slotted spoon.
- ✓ Place the poached egg on top of the avocado toast.
- ✓ Season with salt and pepper and serve.

Greek Yogurt with Berries and Nuts

- 1 cup Greek yogurt, plain
- 1/2 cup mixed berries (strawberries, blueberries, raspberries)
- 1/4 cup nuts (almonds, walnuts)

DIRECTIONS

- ✓ Scoop Greek yogurt into a bowl.
- ✓ Top with fresh berries.
- ✓ Sprinkle nuts over the top.
- ✓ Enjoy a refreshing and protein-rich breakfast.

Protein Pancakes

- 1/2 cup rolled oats
- 1/2 banana
- 1 scoop protein powder
- 2 egg whites
- 1/4 cup almond milk
- 1 tsp baking powder
- 1/2 tsp vanilla extract

DIRECTIONS

- ✓ Blend oats, bananas, protein powder, egg whites, almond milk, baking powder, and vanilla extract until smooth.
- ✓ Heat a non-stick pan and pour batter to form pancakes.
- ✓ Cook until bubbles form on the surface, then flip and cook the other side.

Serve with a dollop of Greek yogurt or fresh fruit.

Smoked Salmon and Avocado Wrap

> ➤ 1 whole-grain tortilla
> ➤ 2 slices smoked salmon
> ➤ 1/2 ripe avocado, sliced
> ➤ 1/4 cup spinach leaves
> ➤ 1 tbsp cream cheese

DIRECTIONS

- ✓ Lay the tortilla flat on a plate.
- ✓ Spread cream cheese over the tortilla.
- ✓ Place smoked salmon, avocado slices, and spinach leaves on top.
- ✓ Roll the tortilla tightly and slice it in half.
- ✓ Serve for a savory, protein-packed breakfast.

Cottage Cheese and Pineapple Bowl

- ➢ 1 cup cottage cheese
- ➢ 1/2 cup pineapple, diced
- ➢ 1 tbsp chia seeds

DIRECTIONS

- ✓ Place cottage cheese in a bowl.
- ✓ Top with diced pineapple.
- ✓ Sprinkle chia seeds over the top.
- ✓ Mix and enjoy this high-protein breakfast.

Veggie Scramble with Quinoa

- ➤ 1/2 cup cooked quinoa
- ➤ 2 eggs
- ➤ 1/4 cup bell peppers, diced
- ➤ 1/4 cup onions, diced
- ➤ 1 tbsp olive oil
- ➤ Salt and pepper to taste

DIRECTIONS

- ✓ Heat olive oil in a pan and sauté onions and bell peppers.
- ✓ Beat eggs and pour into the pan, stirring to scramble.
- ✓ Once the eggs are nearly cooked, stir in the cooked quinoa.
- ✓ Season with salt and pepper and serve warm.

Almond Butter and Banana Smoothie

- 1 banana
- 2 tbsp almond butter
- 1 cup almond milk
- 1 scoop protein powder (optional)
- Ice cubes

DIRECTIONS

- ✓ 1 banana
- ✓ 2 tbsp almond butter
- ✓ 1 cup almond milk
- ✓ 1 scoop protein powder (optional)
- ✓ Ice cubes

Chia Seed Pudding

- ➢ 1/4 cup chia seeds
- ➢ 1 cup almond milk
- ➢ 1/2 tsp vanilla extract
- ➢ 1 tbsp honey or maple syrup
- ➢ Fresh fruit for topping

DIRECTIONS

- ✓ Mix chia seeds, almond milk, vanilla extract, and sweetener in a bowl.
- ✓ Let it sit for 5 minutes, then stir again to prevent clumping.
- ✓ Cover and refrigerate overnight.
- ✓ Top with fresh fruit before serving.

Turkey and Egg Breakfast Muffins

> 4 eggs
> 1/2 cup ground turkey, cooked
> 1/4 cup spinach, chopped
> 1/4 cup bell peppers, diced
> Salt and pepper to taste

DIRECTIONS

- ✓ Preheat oven to 350°F (175°C).
- ✓ Whisk eggs in a bowl and add cooked turkey, spinach, and bell peppers.
- ✓ Season with salt and pepper.
- ✓ Pour mixture into muffin tins and bake for 20-25 minutes.
- ✓ Let cool slightly and serve.

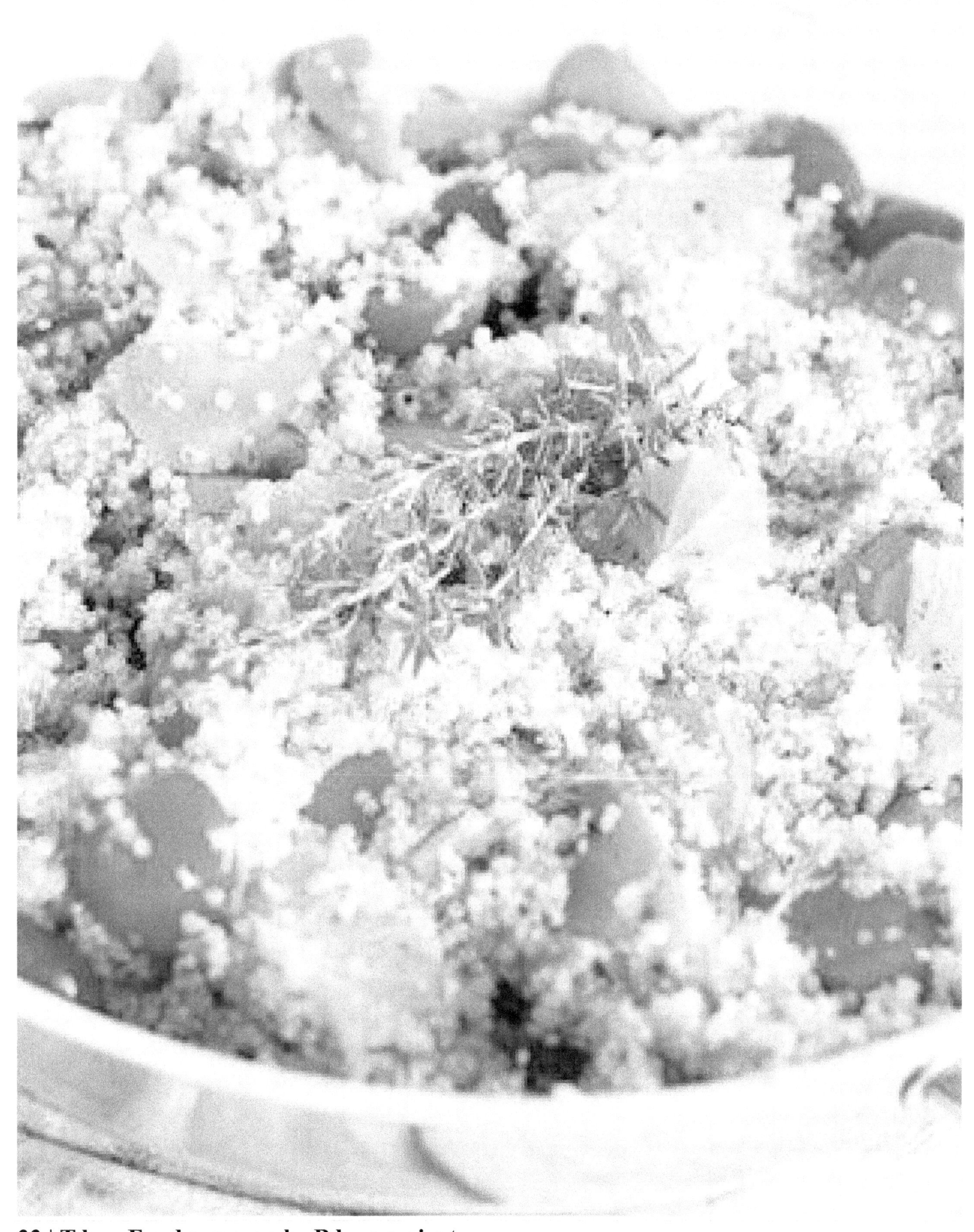

CHAPTER FIVE

LUNCH RECIPES

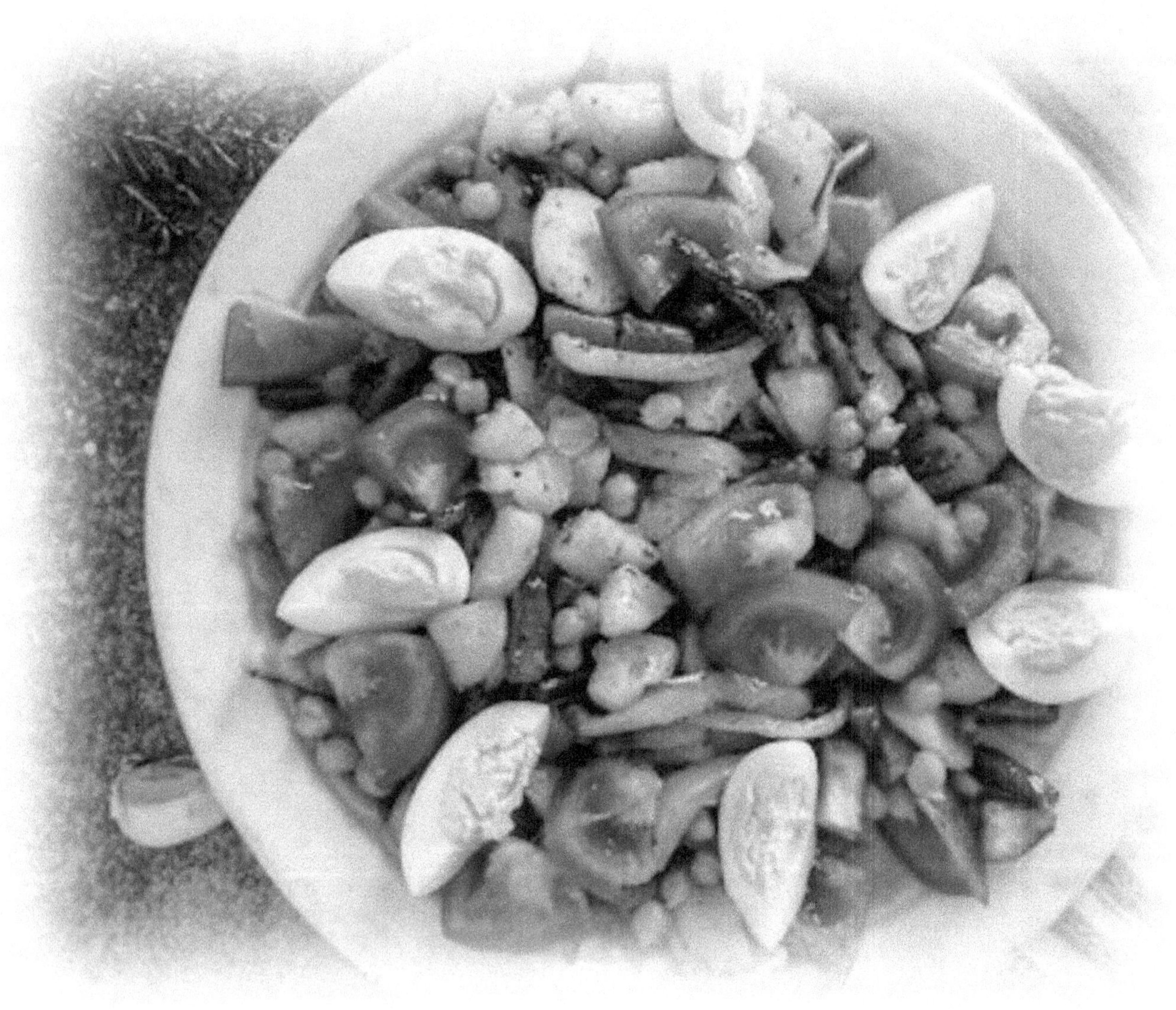

Grilled Chicken Salad

- ➢ 1 chicken breast
- ➢ Mixed greens (lettuce, spinach, arugula)
- ➢ Cherry tomatoes
- ➢ Cucumber
- ➢ Red onion
- ➢ Olive oil
- ➢ Lemon juice
- ➢ Salt and pepper

DIRECTIONS

- ✓ Grill the chicken breast until fully cooked; let it cool and slice.
- ✓ Combine mixed greens, cherry tomatoes, cucumber, and red onion in a bowl.
- ✓ Drizzle with olive oil and lemon juice.
- ✓ Season with salt and pepper.
- ✓ Top with sliced chicken and serve.

Turkey and Quinoa Stuffed Peppers

- ➢ Bell peppers
- ➢ Ground turkey
- ➢ Cooked quinoa
- ➢ Diced tomatoes
- ➢ Garlic powder
- ➢ Onion powder
- ➢ Shredded cheese (optional)
- ➢ Salt and pepper

DIRECTIONS

- ✓ Preheat oven to 375°F (190°C).
- ✓ Brown ground turkey in a pan; season with garlic and onion powder.
- ✓ Mix cooked quinoa and diced tomatoes into the turkey.
- ✓ Cut the tops off the bell peppers and remove the seeds.
- ✓ Stuff peppers with the turkey and quinoa mixture.
- ✓ Top with shredded cheese if desired.
- ✓ Bake for 25-30 minutes until peppers are tender.

Tuna Salad Lettuce Wraps

- ➢ Canned tuna
- ➢ Diced celery
- ➢ Diced red onion
- ➢ Greek yogurt
- ➢ Dijon mustard
- ➢ Lettuce leaves
- ➢ Salt and pepper

DIRECTIONS

- ✓ Mix tuna, celery, red onion, Greek yogurt, and Dijon mustard in a bowl.
- ✓ Season with salt and pepper.
- ✓ Spoon the mixture into lettuce leaves.
- ✓ Roll up and enjoy a light and refreshing lunch.

Lentil Soup

- Lentils
- Carrots
- Celery
- Onion
- Garlic
- Vegetable broth
- Diced tomatoes
- Olive oil
- Thyme
- Salt and pepper

DIRECTIONS

- ✓ Sauté onions, carrots, and celery in olive oil until soft.
- ✓ Add garlic and cook for another minute.
- ✓ Pour in vegetable broth, lentils, and diced tomatoes.
- ✓ Bring to a boil, then simmer until lentils are tender.
- ✓ Season with thyme, salt, and pepper.
- ✓ Serve hot.

Beef and Broccoli Stir-Fry

- ➢ Beef strips
- ➢ Broccoli florets
- ➢ Soy sauce
- ➢ Garlic
- ➢ Ginger
- ➢ Olive oil
- ➢ Sesame seeds

DIRECTIONS

- ✓ Marinate beef strips in soy sauce, garlic, and ginger.
- ✓ Heat olive oil in a pan and stir-fry beef until browned.
- ✓ Add broccoli florets and cook until tender-crisp.
- ✓ Sprinkle with sesame seeds before serving.

Cauliflower Rice Burrito Bowl

- ➢ Cauliflower rice
- ➢ Black beans
- ➢ Corn
- ➢ Avocado
- ➢ Tomato
- ➢ Lime juice
- ➢ Cilantro
- ➢ Salt and pepper

DIRECTIONS

- ✓ Prepare cauliflower rice by pulsing cauliflower in a food processor.
- ✓ Cook cauliflower rice in a pan until tender.
- ✓ Assemble the bowl with cauliflower rice, black beans, corn, diced avocado, and tomato.
- ✓ Drizzle with lime juice and garnish with cilantro.
- ✓ Season with salt and pepper to taste.

Eggplant and Chickpea Stew

- ➢ Eggplant
- ➢ Chickpeas
- ➢ Onion
- ➢ Garlic
- ➢ Diced tomatoes
- ➢ Cumin
- ➢ Paprika
- ➢ Olive oil
- ➢ Salt and pepper

DIRECTIONS

- ✓ Dice eggplant and sauté with onion and garlic in olive oil.
- ✓ Add chickpeas, diced tomatoes, cumin, and paprika.
- ✓ Simmer until eggplant is tender and flavors meld.
- ✓ Season with salt and pepper.
- ✓ Serve warm.

Zucchini Noodle Salad

- Zucchini
- Cherry tomatoes
- Kalamata olives
- Feta cheese
- Olive oil
- Lemon juice
- Salt and pepper

DIRECTIONS

- Spiralize zucchini into noodles.
- Toss zucchini noodles with halved cherry tomatoes, olives, and crumbled feta cheese.
- Dress with olive oil and lemon juice.
- Season with salt and pepper.
- Chill before serving.

Shrimp and Avocado Salad

- ➢ Shrimp
- ➢ Avocado
- ➢ Mixed greens
- ➢ Red onion
- ➢ Olive oil
- ➢ Lemon juice
- ➢ Salt and pepper

DIRECTIONS

- ✓ Cook shrimp in a pan until pink and set aside.
- ✓ Slice avocado and red onion.
- ✓ Toss mixed greens, shrimp, avocado, and onion in a bowl.
- ✓ Dress with olive oil and lemon juice.
- ✓ Season with salt and pepper.

Balsamic Chicken and Veggie Roast

- ➢ Chicken breasts
- ➢ Zucchini
- ➢ Bell peppers
- ➢ Red onion
- ➢ Balsamic vinegar
- ➢ Olive oil
- ➢ Italian seasoning
- ➢ Salt and pepper

DIRECTIONS

- ✓ Preheat oven to 425°F (220°C).
- ✓ Toss chicken and veggies with balsamic vinegar, olive oil, and Italian seasoning.
- ✓ Spread on a baking sheet and roast until chicken is cooked through.
- ✓ Season with salt and pepper.
- ✓ Serve hot.

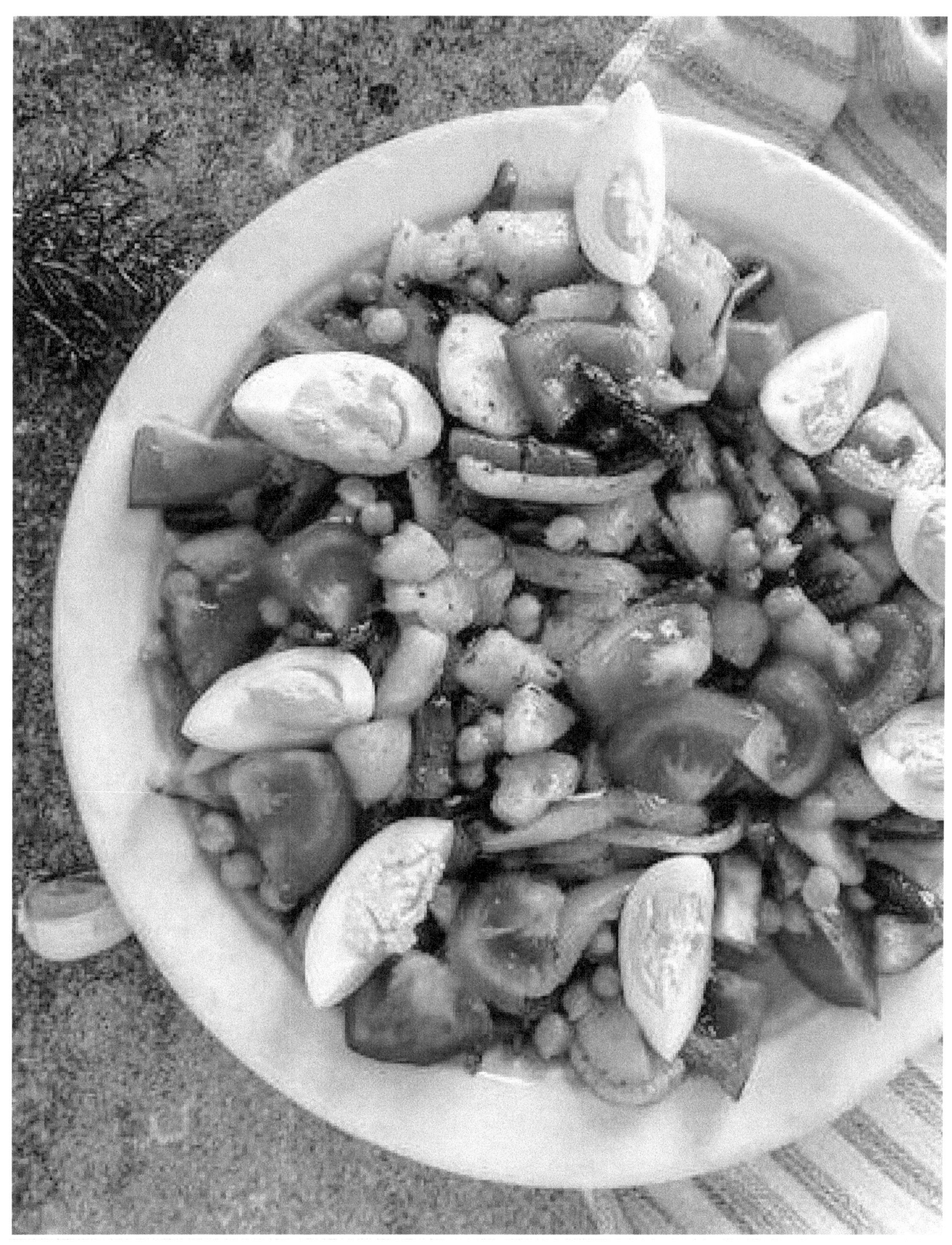

CHAPTER SIX

SNACKS RECIPES

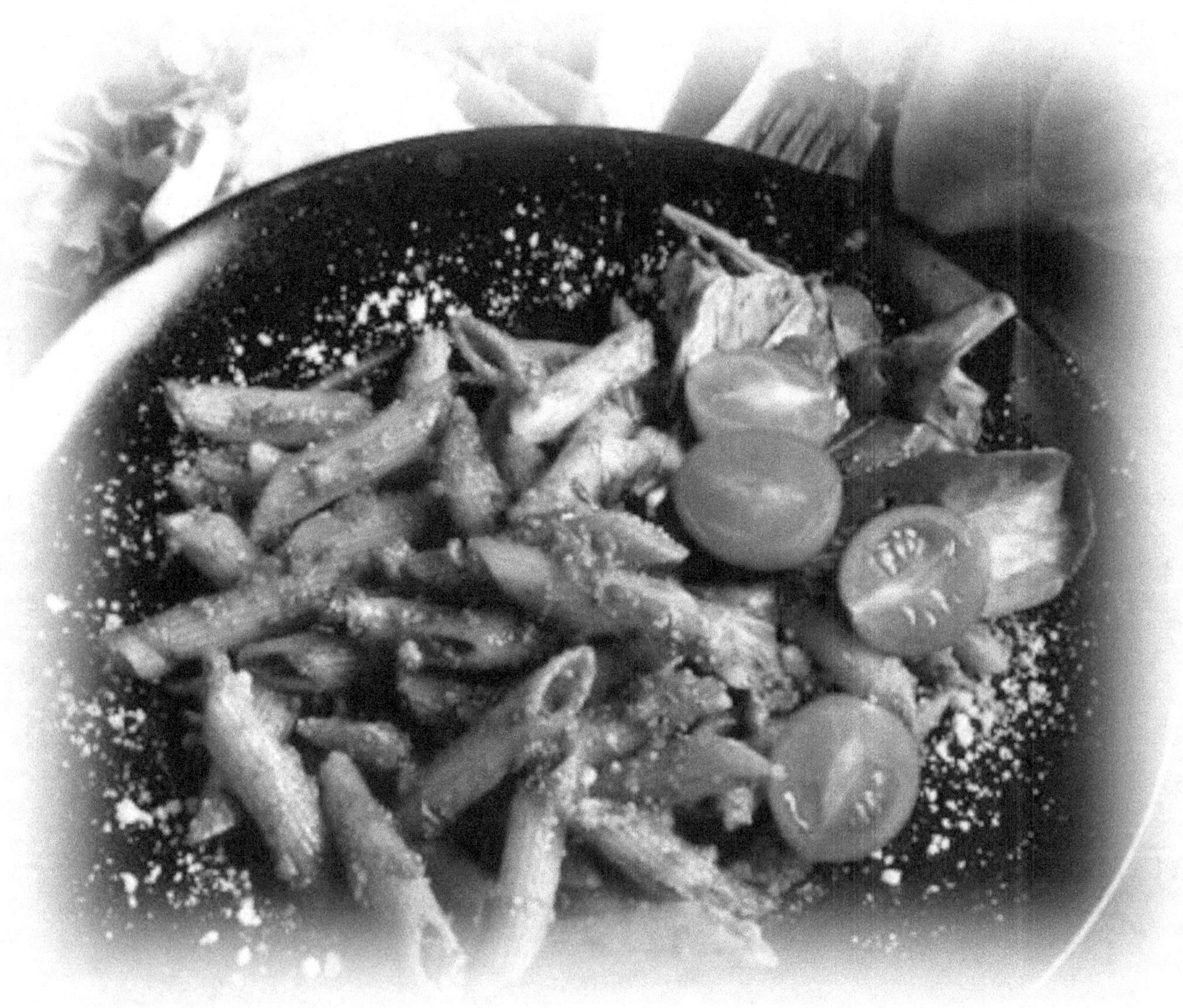

Cucumber Hummus Bites

- ➢ Cucumber slices
- ➢ Hummus
- ➢ Paprika

DIRECTIONS

- ✓ Slice a cucumber into thick rounds.
- ✓ Spread hummus on each cucumber slice.
- ✓ Sprinkle a dash of paprika on top.

Greek Yogurt and Berry Parfait

- Greek yogurt
- Mixed berries (strawberries, blueberries, raspberries)
- A drizzle of honey

DIRECTIONS

- ✓ Layer Greek yogurt and mixed berries in a glass.
- ✓ Drizzle a small amount of honey on top for sweetness.

Almond Butter Celery Sticks

- ➤ Celery sticks
- ➤ Almond butter
- ➤ Raisins

DIRECTIONS

- ✓ Fill the groove of each celery stick with almond butter.
- ✓ Place a few raisins on top of the almond butter.

Turkey Roll-Ups

- ➢ Sliced turkey breast
- ➢ Avocado
- ➢ Spinach leaves

DIRECTIONS

- ✓ Lay out a slice of turkey breast.
- ✓ Place a slice of avocado and a spinach leaf on the turkey.

Roll it up and secure it with a toothpick.

Boiled Egg and Veggie Slices

- ➢ Hard-boiled eggs
- ➢ Sliced bell peppers
- ➢ Sliced cucumbers

DIRECTIONS

- ✓ Peel and slice hard-boiled eggs.
- ✓ Serve with sliced bell peppers and cucumbers.

Cottage Cheese with Pineapple

- ➢ Cottage cheese
- ➢ Diced pineapple

DIRECTIONS

- ✓ Place a scoop of cottage cheese in a bowl.
- ✓ Top with diced pineapple.

Tuna Stuffed Avocado

- ➤ Avocado
- ➤ Canned tuna (drained)
- ➤ Lemon juice
- ➤ Salt and pepper

DIRECTIONS

- ✓ Halve an avocado and remove the pit.
- ✓ Mix tuna with lemon juice, salt, and pepper.
- ✓ Fill the avocado halves with the tuna mixture.

Nutty Yogurt

- ➢ Plain Greek yogurt
- ➢ Chopped nuts (almonds, walnuts)
- ➢ Cinnamon

DIRECTIONS

- ✓ Spoon Greek yogurt into a bowl.
- ✓ Add chopped nuts on top.
- ✓ Sprinkle with cinnamon.

Apple Slices with Peanut Butter

➢ Apple slices
➢ Peanut butter

DIRECTIONS

✓ Core and slice an apple.
✓ Spread peanut butter on each apple slice.

Veggie Chips

- ➢ Thinly sliced vegetables (zucchini, carrots, beets)
- ➢ Olive oil
- ➢ Sea salt

DIRECTIONS

- ✓ Preheat oven to 375°F (190°C).
- ✓ Toss vegetable slices in olive oil and sea salt.
- ✓ Arrange in a single layer on a baking sheet.
- ✓ Bake until crispy, flipping halfway through.

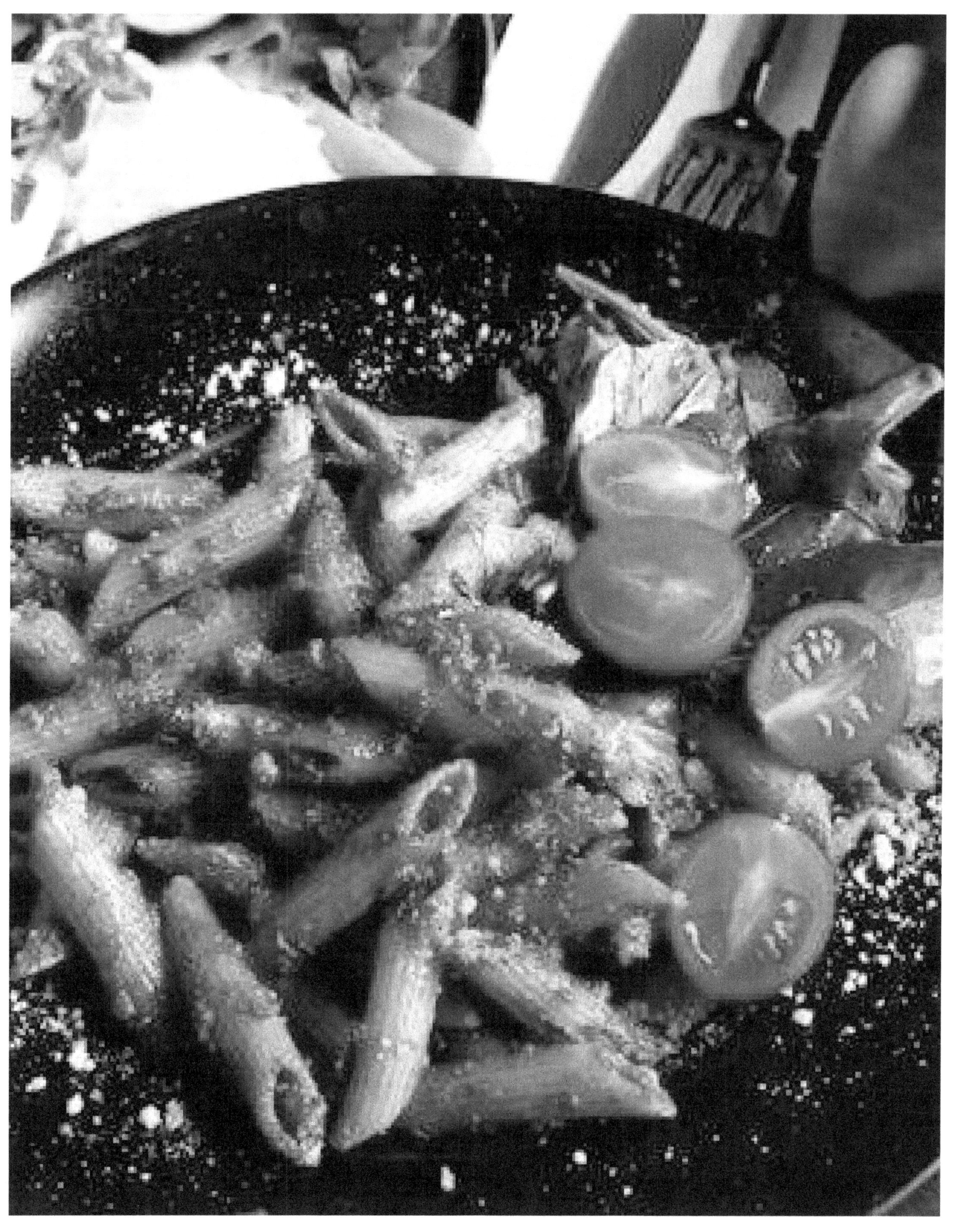

CHAPTER SEVEN

DINNER RECIPES

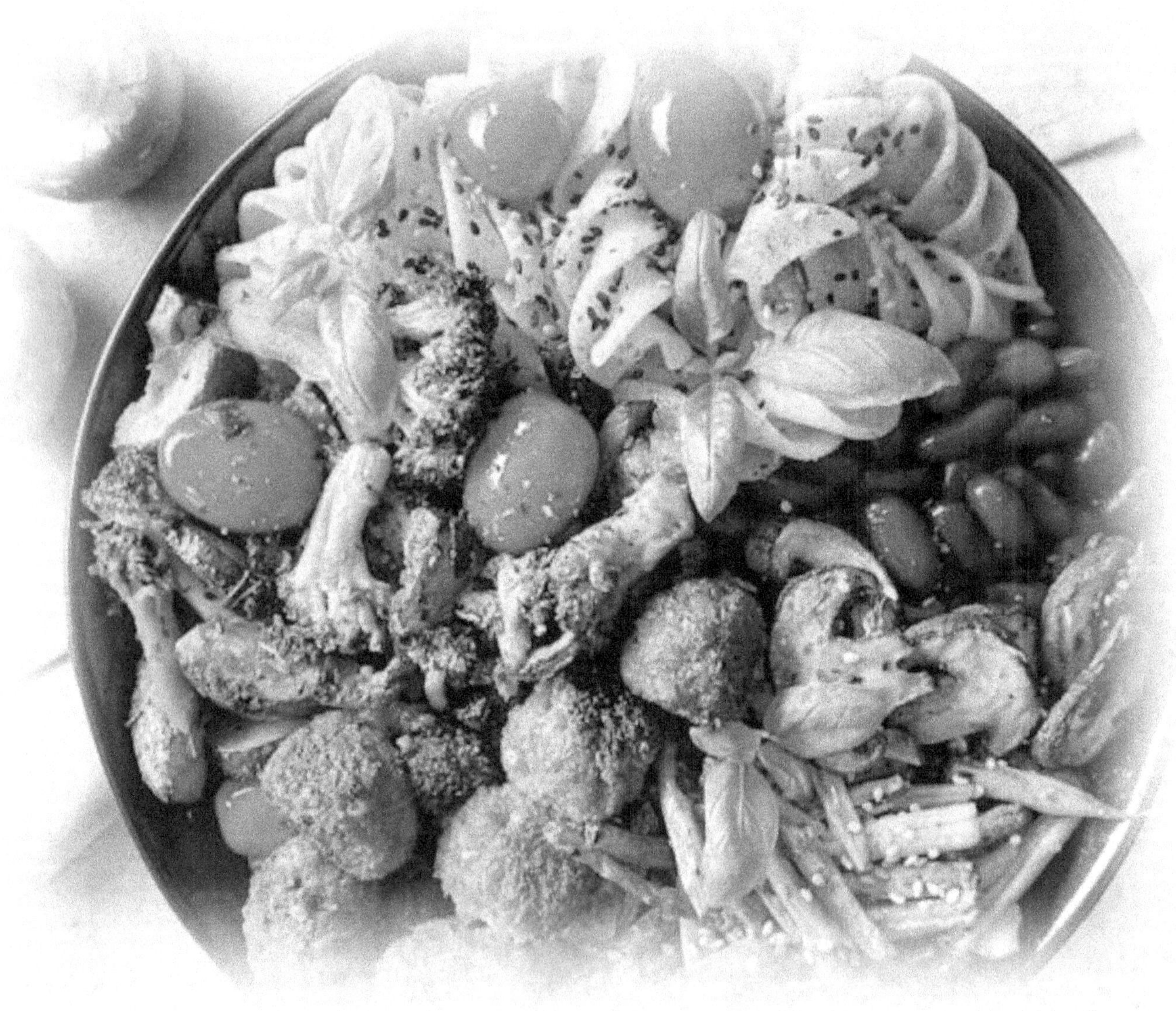

Lemon Herb Grilled Chicken

- ➢ Chicken breasts
- ➢ Lemon juice
- ➢ Olive oil
- ➢ Garlic, minced
- ➢ Fresh herbs (thyme, rosemary, parsley)
- ➢ Salt and pepper

DIRECTIONS

- ✓ Marinate chicken breasts in lemon juice, olive oil, garlic, and herbs.
- ✓ Season with salt and pepper.
- ✓ Grill until cooked through and serve with a side of steamed vegetables.

Baked Salmon with Asparagus

- ➢ Salmon fillets
- ➢ Asparagus spears
- ➢ Olive oil
- ➢ Lemon slices
- ➢ Dill
- ➢ Salt and pepper

DIRECTIONS

- ✓ Place salmon and asparagus on a baking sheet.
- ✓ Drizzle with olive oil and season.
- ✓ Top with lemon slices and dill.
- ✓ Bake until the salmon is flaky.

Turkey Chili

- Ground turkey
- Onion, chopped
- Bell peppers, chopped
- Canned tomatoes
- Kidney beans drained
- Chili powder
- Cumin
- Olive oil
- Salt and pepper

DIRECTIONS

- Sauté onion and bell peppers in olive oil.
- Add ground turkey and cook until browned.
- Stir in tomatoes, beans, and spices.
- Simmer and season to taste.

Stir-fried tofu and Broccoli

- ➢ Firm tofu, cubed
- ➢ Broccoli florets
- ➢ Soy sauce
- ➢ Ginger, grated
- ➢ Garlic, minced
- ➢ Olive oil
- ➢ Sesame seeds

DIRECTIONS

- ✓ Stir-fry tofu in olive oil until golden.
- ✓ Add broccoli, garlic, and ginger.
- ✓ Season with soy sauce and garnish with sesame seeds.

Beef and Vegetable Skewers

- ➢ Beef cubes
- ➢ Zucchini, sliced
- ➢ Bell peppers, chunks
- ➢ Red onion, chunks
- ➢ Olive oil
- ➢ Balsamic vinegar
- ➢ Salt and pepper

DIRECTIONS

- ✓ Thread beef and vegetables onto skewers.
- ✓ Marinate in olive oil and balsamic vinegar.
- ✓ Grill until the beef is cooked to your liking.

Quinoa Stuffed Bell Peppers

- ➢ Bell peppers, halved
- ➢ Cooked quinoa
- ➢ Black beans, drained
- ➢ Corn
- ➢ Tomato, diced
- ➢ Cilantro, chopped
- ➢ Lime juice
- ➢ Salt and pepper

DIRECTIONS

- ✓ Mix quinoa, beans, corn, tomato, and cilantro.
- ✓ Season with lime juice, salt, and pepper.
- ✓ Stuff mixture into bell pepper halves and bake until tender.

Zucchini Noodles with Pesto

- ➢ Zucchini spiralized
- ➢ Basil pesto
- ➢ Cherry tomatoes, halved
- ➢ Pine nuts
- ➢ Parmesan cheese, grated
- ➢ Salt and pepper

DIRECTIONS

- ✓ Toss zucchini noodles with pesto.
- ✓ Add tomatoes and pine nuts.
- ✓ Serve topped with parmesan cheese.

Cauliflower Fried Rice

- ➢ Cauliflower, riced
- ➢ Carrots, diced
- ➢ Peas
- ➢ Egg, beaten
- ➢ Soy sauce
- ➢ Green onions, sliced
- ➢ Olive oil
- ➢ Salt and pepper

DIRECTIONS

- ✓ Sauté carrots and peas in olive oil.
- ✓ Add cauliflower rice and cook until tender.
- ✓ Make a well, add egg, and scramble.
  Season with soy sauce and green onions.

Eggplant Parmesan

- Eggplant, sliced
- Marinara sauce
- Mozzarella cheese, shredded
- Parmesan cheese, grated
- Basil leaves
- Olive oil
- Salt and pepper

DIRECTIONS

- ✓ Roast eggplant slices in olive oil until tender.
- ✓ Layer with marinara sauce and cheese.
- ✓ Bake until bubbly and serve with basil.

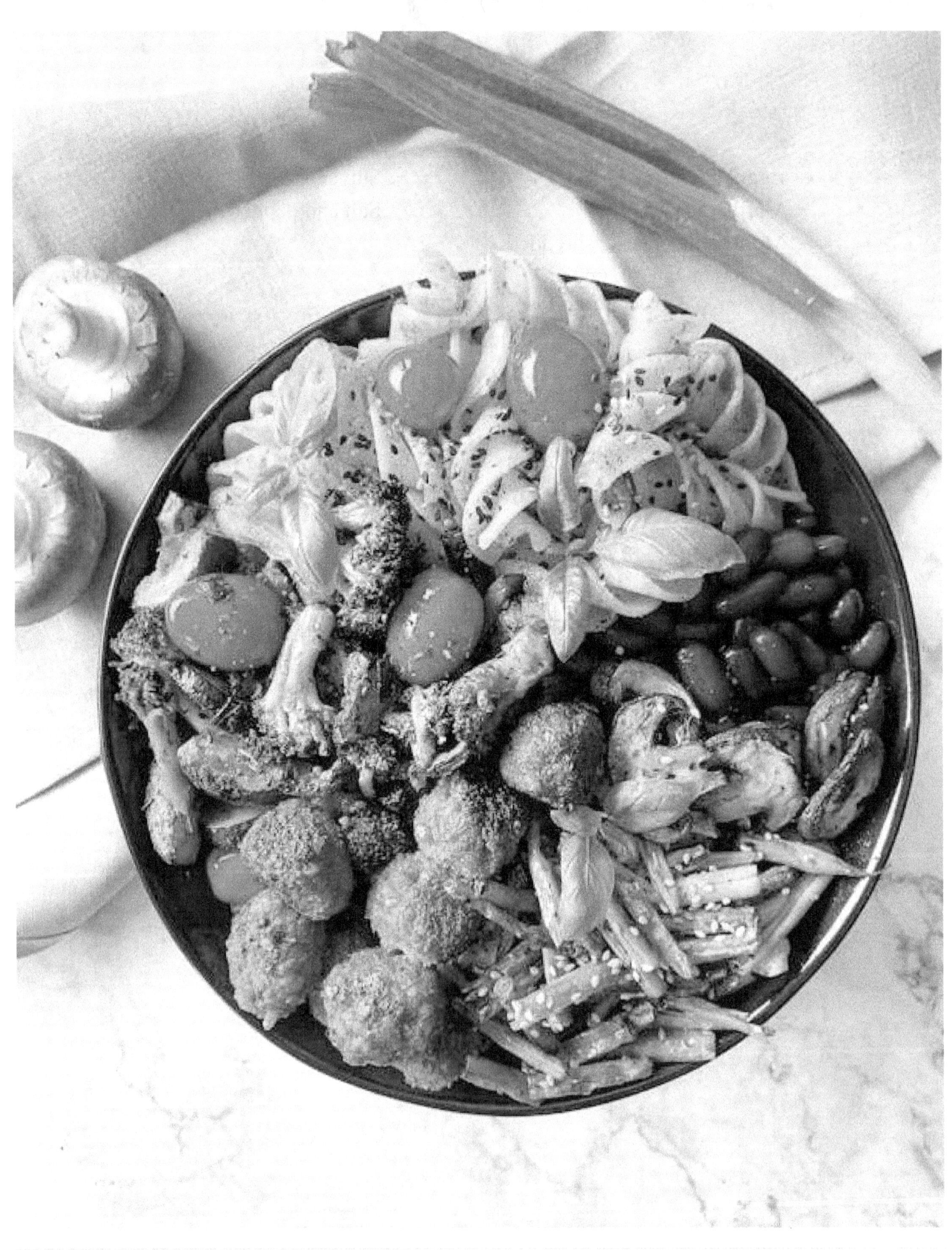

CHAPTER EIGHT: MEAL PLANNING

HOW TO USE THE MEAL PLAN

1. **Understand the Plan:** Review the entire 28-day meal plan to familiarize yourself with the meals and snacks. Note the variety and repetition of certain meals to ensure you're prepared for the upcoming weeks.

2. **Prepare Your Kitchen:** Stock your kitchen with the necessary ingredients for the recipes included in the meal plan. This might involve a weekly grocery shopping trip to ensure freshness, especially for perishable items like vegetables and fruits.

3. **Prep in Advance:** Consider meal prepping at the beginning of the week. Cook and store portions of meals that can be easily reheated or assembled, like grilled chicken, boiled eggs, or chopped vegetables for salads.

4. **Follow the Schedule:** Stick to the daily meal and snack schedule as closely as possible. If you need to swap meals from different days for convenience, try to keep the nutritional balance consistent.

5. **Monitor and Adjust:** Pay attention to how your body responds to the meal plan. If necessary, adjust portion sizes and snack frequency to suit your hunger levels, energy needs, and weight management goals.

Remember, consistency is key, and it's important to stay hydrated and maintain an exercise routine alongside this diet for optimal results. Always consult with a healthcare professional before starting any new diet plan.

28-DAY MEAL PLANS

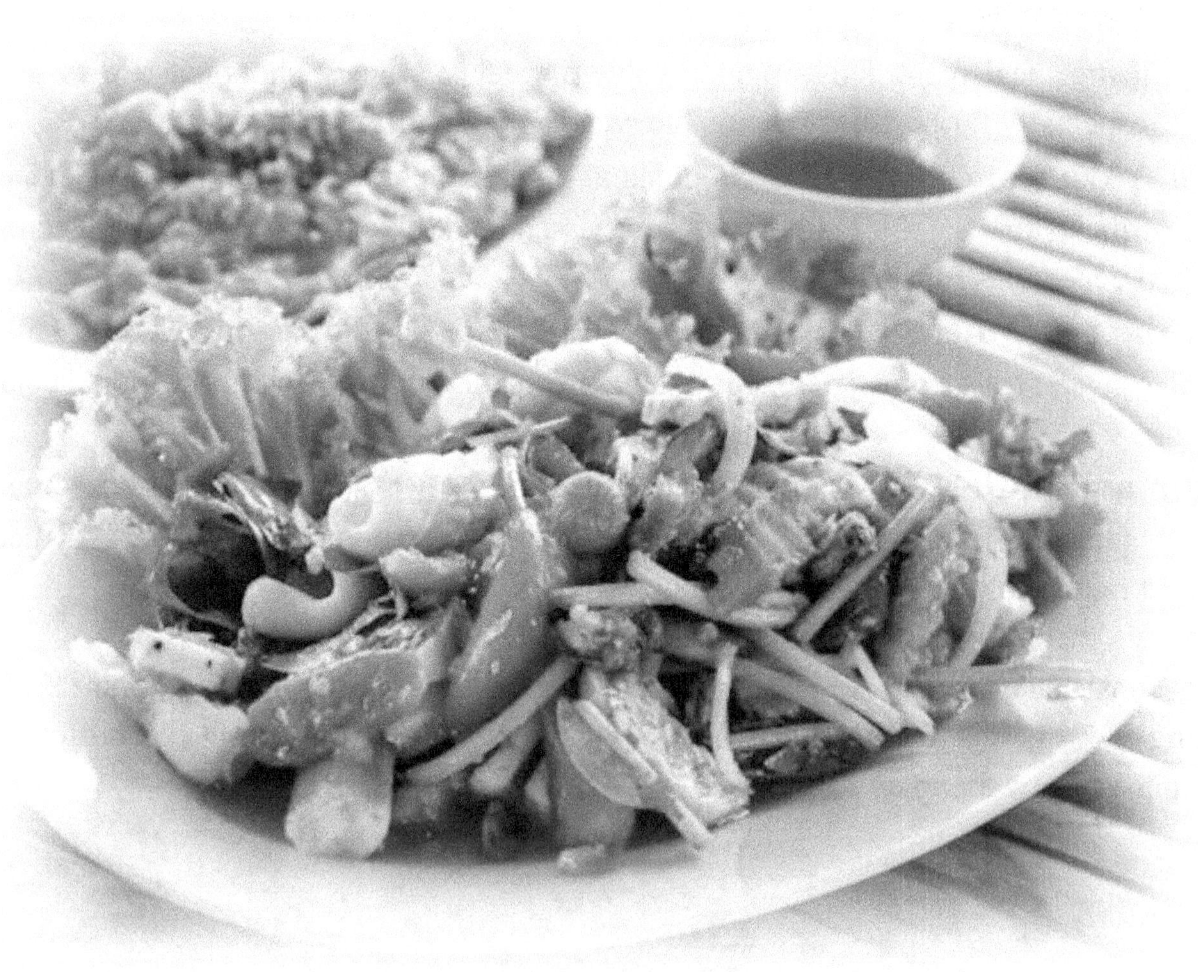

Week 1

MONDAY

BREAKFAST	LUNCH	DINNER	SNACK
Spinach and Mushroom Omelette	Grilled Chicken Salad	Lemon Herb Grilled Chicken	Greek Yogurt and Berry Parfait

TUESDAY

BREAKFAST	LUNCH	DINNER	SNACK
Avocado Toast with Poached Egg	Turkey and Quinoa Stuffed Peppers	Baked Salmon with Asparagus	Turkey Roll-Ups

WEDNESDAY

BREAKFAST	LUNCH	DINNER	SNACK
Greek Yogurt with Berries and Nuts	Tuna Salad Lettuce Wraps	Turkey Chili	Cottage Cheese with Pineapple

THURSDAY

BREAKFAST	LUNCH	DINNER	SNACK
Protein Pancakes	Lentil Soup	Stir-fried tofu and Broccoli	Nutty Yogurt

FRIDAY

BREAKFAST	LUNCH	DINNER	SNACK
Smoked Salmon and Avocado Wrap	Beef and Broccoli Stir-Fry	Veggie Chips	Beef and Vegetable Skewers

SATURDAY

BREAKFAST	LUNCH	DINNER	SNACK
Cottage Cheese and Pineapple Bowl	Cauliflower Rice Burrito Bowl	Quinoa Stuffed Bell Peppers	Cucumber Hummus Bites

SUNDAY

BREAKFAST	LUNCH	DINNER	SNACK
Veggie Scramble with Quinoa	Eggplant and Chickpea Stew	Zucchini Noodles with Pesto	Almond Butter Celery Sticks

Week 2

MEAL PLAN

MONDAY

BREAKFAST	LUNCH	DINNER	SNACK
Almond Butter and Banana Smoothie	Zucchini Noodle Salad	Cauliflower Fried Rice	Cottage Cheese with Pineapple

TUESDAY

BREAKFAST	LUNCH	DINNER	SNACK
Chia Seed Pudding	Shrimp and Avocado Salad	Eggplant Parmesan	Nutty Yogurt

WEDNESDAY

BREAKFAST	LUNCH	DINNER	SNACK
Turkey and Egg Breakfast Muffins	Balsamic Chicken and Veggie Roast	Spicy Shrimp and Kale	Apple Slices with Peanut Butter

THURSDAY

BREAKFAST	LUNCH	DINNER	SNACK
Spinach and Mushroom Omelette	Grilled Chicken Salad	Lemon Herb Grilled Chicken	Greek Yogurt and Berry Parfait

FRIDAY

BREAKFAST	LUNCH	DINNER	SNACK
Avocado Toast with Poached Egg	Turkey and Quinoa Stuffed Peppers	Baked Salmon with Asparagus	Almond Butter Celery Sticks

SATURDAY

BREAKFAST	LUNCH	DINNER	SNACK
Greek Yogurt with Berries and Nuts	Tuna Salad Lettuce Wraps	Turkey Chili	Boiled Egg and Veggie Slices

SUNDAY

BREAKFAST	LUNCH	DINNER	SNACK
Protein Pancakes	Lentil Soup	Stir-fried tofu and Broccoli	Nutty Yogurt

Week 3

MEAL PLAN

MONDAY

BREAKFAST	LUNCH	DINNER	SNACK
Smoked Salmon and Avocado Wrap	Beef and Broccoli Stir-Fry	Beef and Vegetable Skewers	Apple Slices with Peanut Butter

TUESDAY

BREAKFAST	LUNCH	DINNER	SNACK
Cottage Cheese and Pineapple Bowl	Cauliflower Rice Burrito Bowl	Quinoa Stuffed Bell Peppers	Greek Yogurt and Berry Parfait

WEDNESDAY

BREAKFAST	LUNCH	DINNER	SNACK
Veggie Scramble with Quinoa	Eggplant and Chickpea Stew	Zucchini Noodles with Pesto	Turkey Roll-Ups

THURSDAY

BREAKFAST	LUNCH	DINNER	SNACK
Almond Butter and Banana Smoothie	Zucchini Noodle Salad	Cauliflower Fried Rice	Cottage Cheese with Pineapple

FRIDAY

BREAKFAST	LUNCH	DINNER	SNACK
Chia Seed Pudding	Shrimp and Avocado Salad	Eggplant Parmesan	Tuna Stuffed Avocado

SATURDAY

BREAKFAST	LUNCH	DINNER	SNACK
Turkey and Egg Breakfast Muffins	Balsamic Chicken and Veggie Roast	Spicy Shrimp and Kale	Veggie Chips

SUNDAY

BREAKFAST	LUNCH	DINNER	SNACK
Spinach and Mushroom Omelette	Grilled Chicken Salad	Lemon Herb Grilled Chicken	Greek Yogurt Parfait

Week 4

MEAL PLAN

MONDAY

BREAKFAST	LUNCH	DINNER	SNACK
Avocado Toast with Poached Egg	Turkey and Quinoa Stuffed Peppers	Baked Salmon with Asparagus	Almond Butter Celery Sticks

TUESDAY

BREAKFAST	LUNCH	DINNER	SNACK
Greek Yogurt with Berries and Nuts	Tuna Salad Lettuce Wraps	Turkey Chili	Cottage Cheese with Pineapple

WEDNESDAY

BREAKFAST	LUNCH	DINNER	SNACK
Protein Pancakes	Lentil Soup	Stir-fried tofu and Broccoli	Tuna Stuffed Avocado

THURSDAY

BREAKFAST	LUNCH	DINNER	SNACK
Smoked Salmon and Avocado Wrap	Beef and Broccoli Stir-Fry	Beef and Vegetable Skewers	Veggie Chips

FRIDAY

BREAKFAST	LUNCH	DINNER	SNACK
Cottage Cheese and Pineapple Bowl	Cauliflower Rice Burrito Bowl	Quinoa Stuffed Bell Peppers	Cucumber Hummus Bites

SATURDAY

BREAKFAST	LUNCH	DINNER	SNACK
Veggie Scramble with Quinoa	Eggplant and Chickpea Stew	Zucchini Noodles with Pesto	Turkey Roll-Ups

SUNDAY

BREAKFAST	LUNCH	DINNER	SNACK
Almond Butter and Banana Smoothie	Zucchini Noodle Salad	Cauliflower Fried Rice	Boiled Egg and Veggie Slices

CHAPTER NINE: EXERCISE FOR ENDOMORPH

Exercising as an endomorph takes a planned strategy to combat the inherent inclination of this body type to accumulate fat.

Here's how an endomorph should concentrate on exercise:

High-Intensity Interval Training (HIIT)

HIIT is particularly helpful for endomorphs since it burns a considerable quantity of calories in a short time and may enhance insulin sensitivity. This form of training comprises brief bursts of intensive activity followed by rest or low-intensity periods.

Strength Training

Building muscle is crucial for endomorphs since muscular tissue burns more calories than fat, even at rest. Incorporating full-body strength workouts that target all major muscle groups can increase the resting metabolic rate.

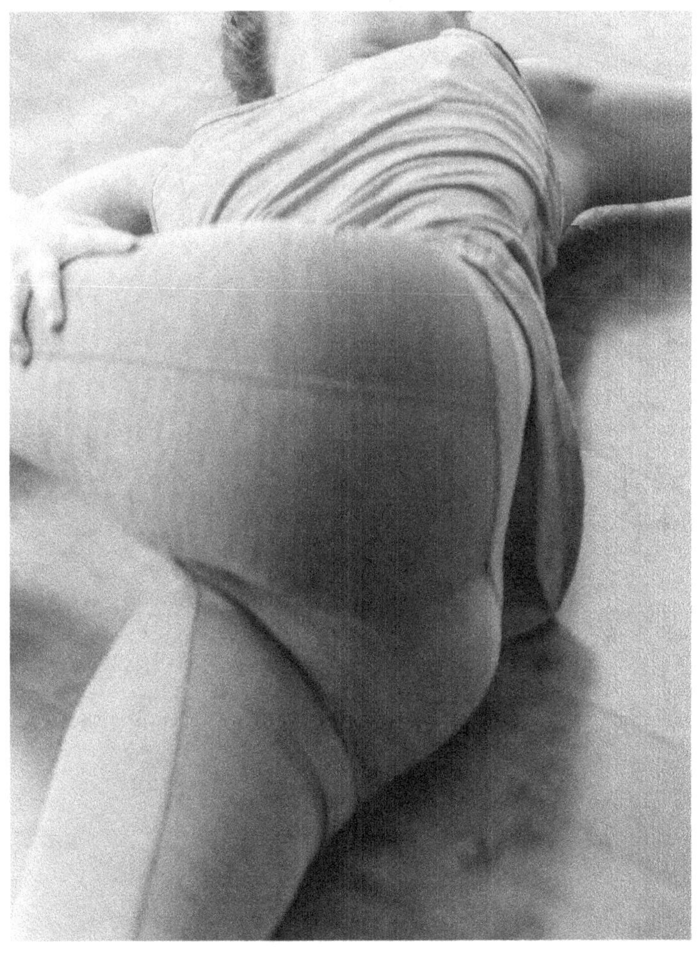

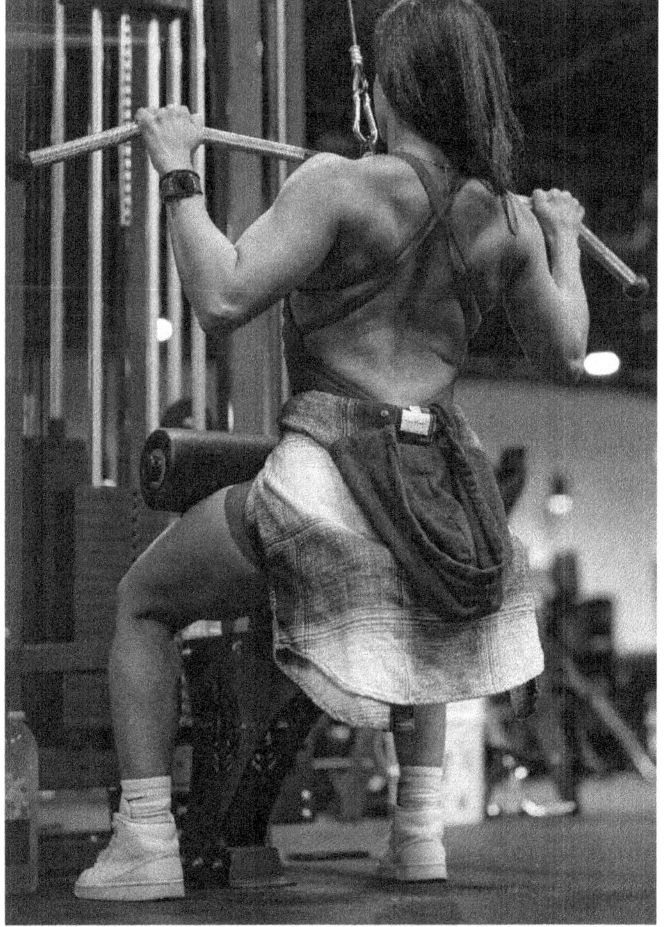

Compound Movements

Exercises that recruit multiple muscle groups, like squats and deadlifts, are beneficial as they lead to higher calorie burn and hormone release that aids in muscle building and fat loss.

Cardiovascular Exercise

In addition to HIIT, steady-state cardio like jogging, cycling, or swimming may aid with fat reduction and cardiovascular health. However, it should not replace strength training but rather complement it.

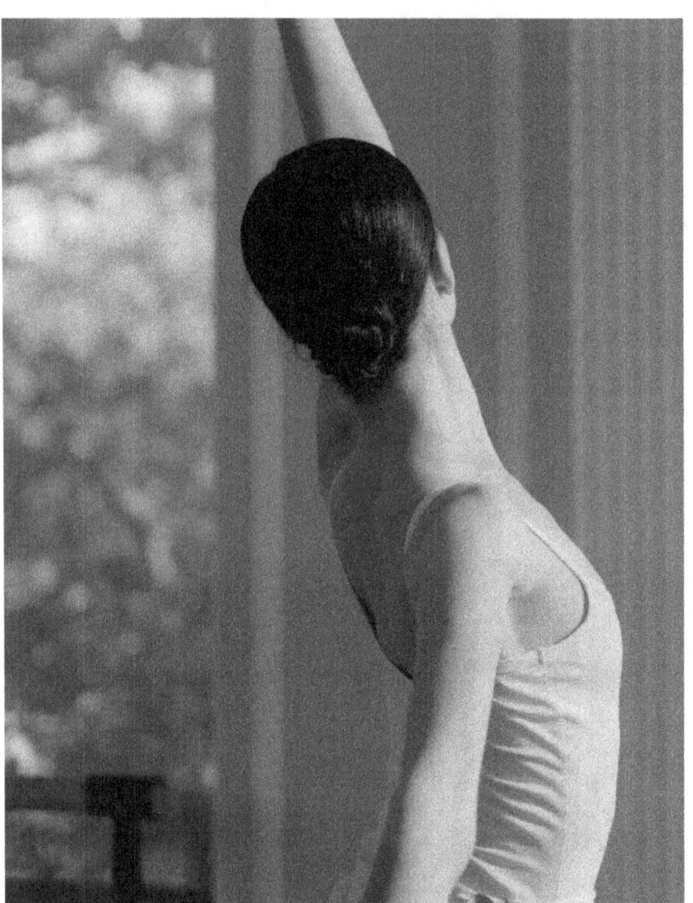

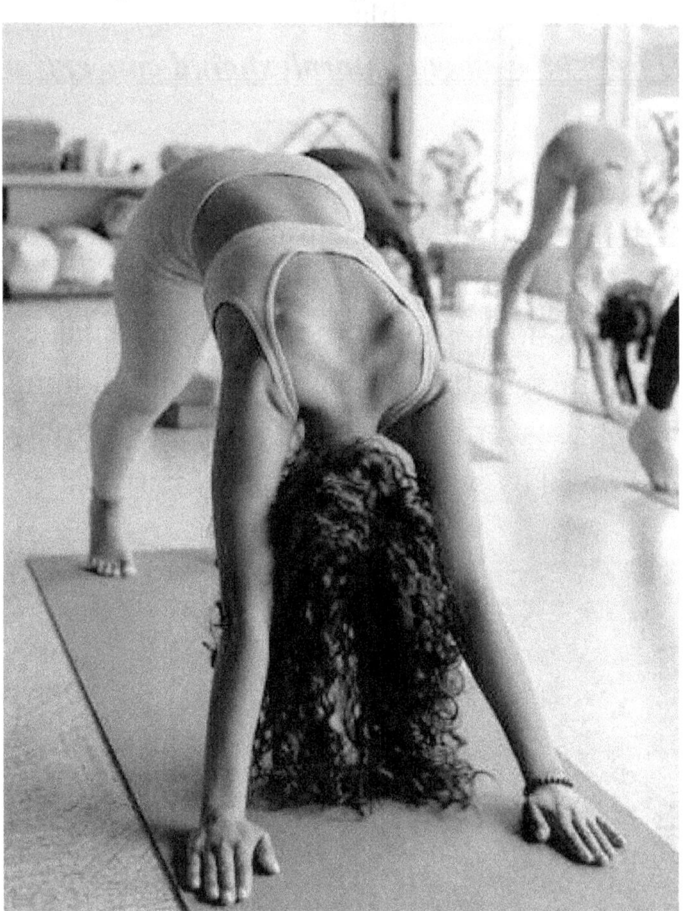

Consistency

Regular exercise is crucial. Endomorphs benefit from going to the gym many times a week, incorporating both weight training and cardio to optimize calorie burn.

By combining these workout routines with a good diet, endomorphs may successfully control their weight and enhance their general fitness. It's vital to start at a comfortable level and gradually build intensity to avoid injury and guarantee long-term commitment to the workout regimen.

CONCLUSION

The Endomorph diet and exercise regimen is a complete method suited to persons with a body type that naturally conserves energy and accumulates fat. This strategy stresses a balanced diet rich in proteins and healthy fats, paired with a targeted exercise schedule that incorporates both strength training and high-intensity interval training (HIIT). The objective is to enhance metabolism, develop lean muscle, and stimulate fat reduction while preserving overall health and vigor.

Adopting this strategy demands attention and perseverance since it entails making smart decisions regarding diet and committing to regular physical exercise. The diet emphasizes full, unprocessed foods that feed the body and promote metabolic function, while the exercise component is aimed to enhance calorie burn and improve body composition.

For people with an endomorphic body type, this strategy is not simply a temporary cure but a lifestyle shift that promotes a healthier, more active way of living. It's about recognizing your body's particular demands and adopting behaviors that will lead to long-term success.

Let this plan be your guide to a changed self. Remember, every step you take is a step towards a healthy you. With each meal and activity, you're not simply reducing weight—you're gaining life. Embrace this path with confidence and persistence, and watch as you uncover the greatest version of yourself. You have the ability to mold your fate; let today be the moment you decide to rise to your greatest potential.

Thank you for reading our endomorph diet for beginners' cookbook. We hope these recipes inspire and guide you on your journey to better health and well-being. Your commitment to making positive changes is commendable, and we wish you great success and enjoyment in every meal you create. Happy cooking!

BONUS: WEEKLY MEAL PLANNER

MEAL PLANNER

	BREAKFAST	LUNCH	DINNER	SNACKS
MON				
TUES				
WED				
THURS				
FRI				
SAT				
SUN				

MEAL PLANNER

	BREAKFAST	LUNCH	DINNER	SNACKS
MON				
TUES				
WED				
THURS				
FRI				
SAT				
SUN				

MEAL PLANNER

	BREAKFAST	LUNCH	DINNER	SNACKS
MON				
TUES				
WED				
THURS				
FRI				
SAT				
SUN				

MEAL PLANNER

	BREAKFAST	LUNCH	DINNER	SNACKS
MON				
TUES				
WED				
THURS				
FRI				
SAT				
SUN				

MEAL PLANNER

	BREAKFAST	LUNCH	DINNER	SNACKS
MON				
TUES				
WED				
THURS				
FRI				
SAT				
SUN				

MEAL PLANNER

	BREAKFAST	LUNCH	DINNER	SNACKS
MON				
TUES				
WED				
THURS				
FRI				
SAT				
SUN				

MEAL PLANNER

	BREAKFAST	LUNCH	DINNER	SNACKS
MON				
TUES				
WED				
THURS				
FRI				
SAT				
SUN				

MEAL PLANNER

	BREAKFAST	LUNCH	DINNER	SNACKS
MON				
TUES				
WED				
THURS				
FRI				
SAT				
SUN				

MEAL PLANNER

	BREAKFAST	LUNCH	DINNER	SNACKS
MON				
TUES				
WED				
THURS				
FRI				
SAT				
SUN				

MEAL PLANNER

	BREAKFAST	LUNCH	DINNER	SNACKS
MON				
TUES				
WED				
THURS				
FRI				
SAT				
SUN